Snore Wars! is a MUST read foi
deal and thanks to him I unde
and the lives of many others, sle
explained in the book. Thank yo

Colin G. Dobbins, patient for over 10 years

As a sufferer of Obstructive Sleep Apnoea for over 15 years I read this book with great interest. Oko is a master of his craft and his clean and concise analysis on the causes of sleep apnoea and the various treatments available. Shockingly, there are over four million sufferers in the UK – the figures are mind blowing making this book a must read. He highlights the huge economic, personal and social costs. His incisive observations and recommendations face the sleep apnoea future with confidence. This is a wake-up call for anyone who snores and their partners. As he aptly states 'Sleep is the best medicine'.

Mike Tanousis, current patient

SNORE WARS!

If SNORING is ruining your nights, here's how to win the day

DR MICHAEL OKO

First published in Great Britain by Practical Inspiration Publishing, 2025

© Michael Oko, 2025

The moral rights of the author have been asserted

ISBN   9781788607247   (hardback)
       9781788607254   (paperback)
       9781788607278   (epub)
       9781788607261   (Kindle)

Every effort has been made to trace copyright holders and to obtain their permission for the use of copyright material. The publisher apologizes for any errors or omissions and would be grateful if notified of any corrections that should be incorporated in future reprints or editions of this book.

Want to bulk-buy copies of this book for your team and colleagues? We can customize the content and co-brand *Snore Wars!* to suit your business's needs.

Please email info@practicalinspiration.com for more details.

Practical Inspiration
Publishing

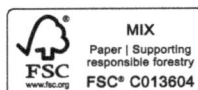

MIX
Paper | Supporting responsible forestry
FSC
www.fsc.org   FSC® C013604

Contents

About the author

Mr Oko is a consultant ENT Surgeon with a special interest and expertise in sleep apnoea and other sleeping disorders. He qualified in 1986 and trained at St Mary's Hospital, London, and Royal National Throat, Nose and Ear Hospital, London. He was a lecturer at the University of Glasgow in ENT surgery and was one of the 12 finalists in 1995 for the Surgeon in Training medal for instrument design and innovation.

Since 2005, he has worked as a Consultant ENT Surgeon within the United Lincolnshire Hospitals Trust (ULHT). In 2006, he founded the Snoring Disorders Centre based at Pilgrim Hospital in Boston at the request of the Medical Director and Consultant Respiratory Physician Dr David Boldy as there was a desperate need for a service in Lincolnshire.

Lincolnshire had the most obese population in Europe and patients had a 4-hour round trip to Nottingham, Leicester or Cambridge to get treatment. He opened satellite clinics, including one in Harley Street, London. His revolutionary sleep service at ULHT won the NHS East Midlands Healthcare Award for service transformation.

In 2013, he worked as an advisor on OSA for the Department of Health. He transformed his service again in 2020 when the COVID-19 pandemic hit. He moved all of his 5,000 patients onto a virtual platform to deliver remote consultations, home sleep studies, home installations of

CPAP machines and masks. These patients had Wi-Fi enabled CPAP devices that could be remotely reset and controlled avoiding unnecessary attendances in the hospital or at home.

COVID-19 was a terrifying experience for many patients and clinicians, but none more so than OSA patients with already-impaired breathing. COVID-19 remains prevalent within the population, so for vulnerable patients such as OSA-sufferers there is a major clinical benefit in avoiding unnecessary hospital attendances where remote treatment provides an appropriate and adequate alternative. This is most apparent for routine follow-up appointments for CPAP-compliant patients – in 80% there is absolutely no reason to expose such patients to the risk of hospital-acquired COVID-19. We note from the following report at https://pubmed. ncbi.nlm.nih.gov/32989673/ that:

'Patients with OSA experienced approximately eight times greater risk for COVID-19 infection compared to a similar age population receiving care in a large, racially, and socioeconomically diverse healthcare system. Among patients with COVID-19 infection, OSA was associated with increased risk of hospital-ization and approximately double the risk of developing respiratory failure.'

It is estimated that between 95,000 and 167,000 patients contracted COVID-19 in England's hospitals during the period from June 2020 to March 2021 alone (www.bmj.com/content/383/bmj.p2399). COVID-19 is of course far from the only potential hospital-acquired infection or disease. A resent UK meta-analysis has shown that virtual consultations are as effective as face-to-face for the management of sleep apnoea.[1]

In 2023, he became a founding member of the All-Parliamentary Working Group (APPG) to advise the House of Lords and Parliament on sleep apnoea and represents with Prof Ram Dhillon ENTUK in this forum. With the new Governments shift in funding to community and home-based services this model of delivery is something Wes Streeting should really be looking at as a quick win!

After his wife complained about his snoring, Dr Oko was diagnosed with moderate sleep apnoea, and he uses the same treatment he prescribes to his patients.

Acknowledgements

Iwould like to thank my wife Lucy for all her support through my long and all-consuming career, and my children, Chantelle, Cameron, India and Joshua for all the times I have been at work and not been with them.

Special thanks go to Dr David Boldy, former Medical Director at United Lincolnshire Hospitals Trust, and Professor Ram Dhillon, my long-term friend and clinical partner in developing sleep services.

Foreword

It is a rare and remarkable feat to take a subject so deeply entrenched in our daily lives, yet often overlooked, and transform it into something both captivating and enlightening. In *Snore Wars!*, Dr Michael Oko has done just that. As a leading expert in sleep disorders, Dr Oko merges his profound clinical knowledge with an engaging narrative that is as informative as it is delightfully entertaining.

From the very first pages, *Snore Wars!* pulls you into the world of sleep, where the nightly symphonies of snoring become not just a matter of health, but a reflection of personal stories, relationships and the uncharted territories of human biology. Dr Oko, with his extraordinary talent for storytelling, invites readers to embark on a journey that explores the science of sleep with clarity, humour and an unshakable sense of curiosity.

What makes *Snore Wars!* truly special, however, is not just the impeccable research or the accessible way it is presented. It is Dr Oko's ability to weave a narrative that is both personal and universal. He manages to balance the seriousness of his medical expertise with a light-hearted approach that makes this book not only educational but thoroughly enjoyable.

As someone who has observed firsthand the transformative power of addressing sleep disorders, Dr Oko has penned a work that could truly change lives. Whether you're someone affected by snoring, or simply intrigued by the mysteries of sleep, *Snore Wars!* offers something for everyone – a fascinating, insightful and often amusing guide into a world most of us never think to explore.

It is my great pleasure to introduce this important work. *Snore Wars!* will not only enlighten but, perhaps, provide the key to a better night's sleep for many. Dr Michael Oko has created a brilliant and necessary contribution to the field of sleep medicine, and I wholeheartedly commend this book to you.

Lord Peter Cruddas

Introduction

Why I have written this book

This book can save your relationship, your sanity or even your life. That's a bold claim but as a leading UK sleep apnoea specialist, it's one I stand by.

This book is for my current and future patients to help them truly understand the condition and why it's so important to use your treatment.

Sleep apnoea is one of the most dangerous and least understood of sleep disorders. But it's one everyone should be talking about, not least because its main symptom causes the biggest battle in the bedroom: snoring. Around 38% of men and 30% of women snore at night and one in five of those snorers will have sleep apnoea.[2]

Apnoea is the temporary cessation of breathing, hence no oxygen gets into your body, and your brain and heart are particularly sensitive. That's serious. It affects the whole body and is a (not-so-) silent epidemic. Yet only 10% of people with this deadly condition currently get diagnosed. So that means over four million people in the UK go to bed every night not knowing they have sleep apnoea. And that's a conservative estimate! That's a lot of people driving their partners mad with loud snoring and facing horrendous health consequences.

By the time many of our patients arrive at the Snore Disorders Centre they're in a state of desperation. Many feel depressed, exhausted and struggle with everything including their work, families and relationships.

All of them will have tried other remedies or seen other doctors. Most of my patients are men in their 50s and 60s. Many have been dragged to the sleep clinic appointment by partners or wives. However, 40% of my sleep clinic patients are women and we also treat children. Regular comments I hear include:

'Doc, if you can't sort him out, we're divorcing.'

'He wakes up making terrible gasping sounds.'

'He's always so grumpy every morning, we don't know what's wrong!'

'She snores like a pig but doesn't like me saying.'

'I stay awake listening for the next breath, worrying it's the last.'

'Even our dog is even traumatized by the noise!'

That anecdote about the dog always raises a few snorts of laughter. And maybe it *is* funny, unless you are the dog… or the snorer's partner. Many other people can't find anything funny about snoring at all.

We should all aim to spend one third of our lives asleep. If we don't sleep properly (either by not getting enough hours or sleeping deeply enough), its impact is devastating on the other two thirds of our life. Lack of sleep affects how we function: physically, mentally and emotionally.

If you regularly do not sleep for the recommended 7–8 hours, then your health *will* certainly suffer. Sleep apnoea and poor sleep is linked with high blood pressure, cardiovascular disease, diabetes, immune diseases, dementia, cancer, brain fog, depression and anxiety.

The stark reality is this. Those with untreated severe sleep apnoea have a staggering 30% chance of a stroke and a 15% chance of cardiac arrest within 12 years. Suddenly loud snoring is even less amusing. If we want to save lives and prevent many chronic illnesses, everyone should understand sleep apnoea.

The battle to make everyone aware of sleep apnoea begins in the bedroom. It often starts with one angry sleep deprived partner. The snorer might react defensively or get sent to the spare room before the following night's skirmish. The fact is, if you have sleep apnoea, no snoring 'remedy' will work. You need proper investigations and treatment.

But how can this war be won? This is where *Snore Wars!* steps in.

This book is divided into four parts. Part one, *'Understanding sleep and snoring'* explains the science behind deep sleep. Why do our bodies need sleep? What is the difference between 'ordinary' snoring and 'sleep apnoea' snoring?

Part two, *'Snore wars!'* examines the different ways men and women react to snoring and seeking treatment. While men tend to ignore the snore, women are often the health gatekeeper for loved ones and themselves! At the Snoring Disorders Centre, we are often the final frontier. But how do you persuade a reluctant partner to get a sleep test in the first place? Included in this section is a specialist questionnaire to assess if someone might have sleep apnoea.

Part three, '*A mad, tired world*' is a deep dive into why society and culture doesn't value sleep and the cost to us all. Understanding this helps us fight back to get the sleep we need.

Part four, '*Sleep, the best medicine*' examines finding the easiest pathway to help. Sleep apnoea can be cured on the NHS with simple treatments but navigating the route can be a minefield. In a step-by-step guide, I make it easy, even for the most reluctant of patients.

We end the book with a section busting common sleep myths and my manifesto for bringing sleep apnoea into the public consciousness.

Understanding sleep apnoea and stopping snoring needn't be a battle. This book can act as a peace treaty for anyone who snores, anyone driven mad by snoring or parents of a child who snores.

It's time to wake up to sleep apnoea.

Dr Michael Oko, July 2024

Part one

Understanding sleep and snoring

Chapter one

The new science behind sleep

Sleep is an essential function to human life but why we sleep remains a mystery. Theories suggest we evolved to sleep because our inert bodies are less vulnerable to predators or because we are less likely to find food at night. But growing scientific evidence reveals sleep is necessary to recharge and regenerate our bodies.

In one study compared to our closest primate relatives, human beings were found to sleep less but more deeply.[3] The incredible efficiency of human sleep could be why we evolved to become the species we are today. However, busy modern lives threaten this uber efficient sleep window. Sleep disorders – like sleep apnoea – make this restorative opportunity shrink even further.

The effects of lack of proper sleep are cumulative too. We can't 'catch up' on sleep. We need to make sure the sleep we have is regular and deep. This is because sleeping is not a passive process. In fact, what happens after we fall asleep is an extraordinarily active process.

The glymphatic system

'Sleep is when all the unsorted stuff comes flying out as from a dustbin upset in a high wind.'

William Golding[4]

After a poor night's sleep, we feel hellish but what is lack of sleep doing to our body and our long-term health? Let's start with the brain.

In terms of weight the brain makes up for just 2% of volume of our bodies, but it consumes a massive 24–28% of all calories we ingest. I imagine the brain to be like a giant raging furnace in a factory, powering everything we say, think and process when we're awake.

Just like in a real factory's furnace, our brain creates waste products after using energy (in this case, oxygen and glucose). A clean-up process is necessary in every metabolic process so why should it be any different for the brain?

The process of sleep is therefore like the bin men coming around to remove daytime junk so you can wake up feeling clean and fresh. If you compare an EEG (electroencephalogram, which records brain activity) of someone who is awake to someone who is in REM sleep, it shows a similar amount of brain activity. In fact, at times, the person who is asleep exhibits 20% to 30% more brain activity in different regions.

Science backs up this theory. One of the most recent discoveries is the 'glymphatic system' which is a waste clearance system formed by specific cells to eliminate soluble proteins and metabolites – waste products of our metabolism.

Incredibly, the glymphatic system was only discovered in 2013, by a Danish neuroscientist called Maiken Nedergaard. This discovery highlights how sleep science really is the Cinderella of medicine. The science behind sleep, such a basic function has been virtually ignored, when it is considered how surgery has been around since 1505 (with the Foundation of The Royal College of Surgeons Edinburgh by King James IV) and funding for sleep apnoea has only been since 2008!

The name 'glymphatic' refers to the glial cells, vital to waste clearance that works in a similar way to the lymphatic system, which clears waste from our nervous system. Glial cells nourish and protect our neurons, the brain cells that send and receive information.

The brain also produces toxic waste including Tau proteins and Amyloid Beta aggregates which cause damage if they build up and are not flushed away. A bit like plaque building up on our teeth which results in tooth decay. If we don't sleep, our brain backs up like a blocked toilet hence brain fog and confusion. Another way of thinking about it is 'cerebral constipation' as we all understand what gut constipation feels like! Unpleasant, sluggish and full of toxins.

There is evidence that if this build-up is not removed it leads to neurodegenerative diseases such as Alzheimer's disease, the most common form of dementia.[5]

High blood pressure and sleep

Nedergaard and her team, made discoveries about how high blood pressure affects the glymphatic system on mice. The effectiveness of the glymphatic system relies on the blood pumping from the arterial wall but high blood pressure stiffens arteries, making it harder to clear the toxins away.

They noticed high blood pressure prevented the clearance of big molecules such as beta-amyloid which is linked to dementia. Several studies have already linked high blood pressure to dementia and so the glymphatic system could be this missing link![6]

Essentially the glymphatic system only wakes up and starts working when we're deeply asleep. This unique function simply doesn't work when we're awake. There is no way of replicating this cleansing process either, such as taking a sleeping pill or meditating or trying any other form of rest.

We must sleep and sleep deeply or we don't get the rubbish cleared out. Simple as that. It then follows if you don't sleep well for most of your life, in my opinion, you're highly likely to develop dementia.

Sleep fact: If you live to average age of 83 in the UK, that mean you should have enjoyed 27 years of sleep!

What exactly is 'deep sleep'?

We all know what it feels like to wake up from a good night's sleep (or at least have a memory of this!). We open our eyes, without the need for an alarm to jolt us awake. We feel clear headed, refreshed, energetic and enjoy an optimistic mood. Life feels good.

If we don't sleep well our body aches, our eyes feel strained, we feel irritable, moody, easily overwhelmed. This leaves our ability to face the challenges of the day severely diminished.

If anyone asks the question: 'Did you sleep well last night?' we can give an instinctive response without really thinking about it. It's either a yes or a no. But how do we achieve this deep restorative sleep? What kind of sleep is necessary for the glymphatic system to work properly? This where we need to understand the sleep cycle, including NREM (non-rapid eye movement) and REM (rapid eye movement).

Explaining the Zzzzzz cycle

Here is a deep dive into the sleep cycle broken down into four stages. We need to experience every single stage in order to revitalize and repair our bodies.

We talk about two broad types of sleep REM and non-REM

Non-REM is divided into light and deep sleep, where we spend about 50% and 25% of our night respectively.

Non-REM cycle

Stage one: Light sleep

Non-REM is 'non-rapid eye movement' and the first stage of which is where our brainwaves, heartbeat and muscle activity all slows down. We often think of this part as 'dozing off'. You're not completely asleep, but not awake either.

It's at this stage we can experience muscle twitches, where the body jerks unexpectedly, some of which we can be aware of as we sink into a sleep. Sometimes if you wake from this stage, it feels like you weren't asleep at all, this is because the brain is still active. You may feel semi-conscious and like you were half-asleep: 'I'm not snoring – I was awake!' the snorer laments when challenged in this stage.

People who suffer from insomnia can often feel 'stuck' in this first dozing stage and feel frustrated when they don't move onto the next stage, the part where you really dive into the pool of sleep.

Sometimes jerking muscles alarms people, and the worse thing is, increased tiredness makes muscles jerk more. Sometimes being conscious of the need to sleep is enough to cause hesitation in allowing ourselves to drift to the next stage. We deal with insomnia later in the book.

The length of this first cycle lasts around 5 to 10 minutes.

Stage two: Light sleep

Stage two of NREM involves the heart, breathing and body temperature all decreasing. This is where the brain waves change to distinct patterns called 'sleep spindles' where activity in the brain makes short spikes of higher frequency brainwaves, thought to be important for learning.

Short bursts of electrical activity also occur called K-complexes. Both activities are thought to help a person process their memories of the previous intake of information.

This is why it's important to get a good night's sleep if we're learning something new the next day. We need a good night's sleep the day after too, for the memories to embed.

This period of sleeping makes up for about 50% of the total time we are asleep.

The length of this cycle can be 10 to 25 minutes.

Stage three: Deep sleep

Stage three of NREM is where we sink deeper into the pool of a deep, restorative sleep. I call this the 'siren' sleep, because it's the deep pool of sleep that keeps on tempting sleepers in.

It's where slow, lower frequency 'Delta' brainwaves take over, and breathing decreases further, blood pressure lowers. If someone tries to wake us up at this point, we'd feel groggy and be difficult to wake.

This stage of sleep is vital when it comes to repairing our bodies. It's where cell regeneration occurs, including tissue repairs and growth. It's where our immune system is strengthened. It's also when our all-important glymphatic system wakes up and kicks in. This part of the cycle cleans the debris in our brain.

The length of this cycle is 20 to 40 minutes.

The REM cycles

The final stage of the sleep cycle is the REM, rapid eye movement. This is when eye movements move rapidly from left to right and brain activity hugely increases along with breathing and heart rate. Dreams occur in this stage, but our bodies become paralyzed, so we don't start acting out what is happening in the dream. At each cycle the REM length gets longer, so for the first round it could be 10 minutes, the second round 30 minutes and the third round 60 minutes.

On average an adult should experience three to five rounds of REM. The ideal goal is to experience 90 minutes in total of REM, which is achievable with 8 hours sleep.

Those who snore persistently or have sleep apnoea often miss out on this deep REM part of the cycle.

If you don't get enough REM sleep, you will know about it. This is because you will feel groggy, forgetful, irritable, have trouble focusing and feel tired. You're also more likely to be hungry because the lack of REM causes a spike in the hormone ghrelin, which causes hunger. It also causes the hormone Leptin to decrease, which is the hormone that makes you feel full up. That's why when we're overtired, we crave food, and nothing feels satiating.

This double whammy is why tired people are far more likely to choose high sugar, high fat foods, calorific foods and why poor sleepers tend to pile on weight.

All sleep stages do not occur in order necessarily, but the REM is the final stage of the cycles and typically, the stage of REM increases as the night goes on. You should enjoy three to five rounds, the last being between the hours of 5am and 7am if you're reaching the golden 8 hours sleep.

We're often in the last cycle between 6am and 7am, which is why people can feel pretty peeved at the alarm clock going off!

Be mindful too that alcohol, certain antidepressants, marijuana and caffeine are all substances which suppress REM sleep.

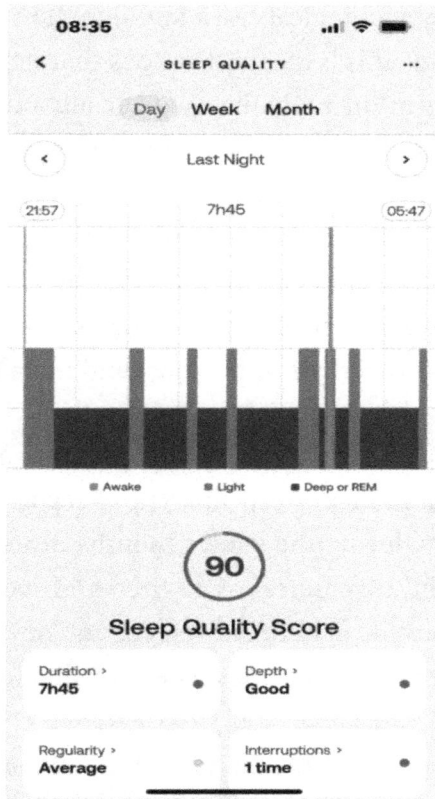

Figure 1.1 Screenshot of App showing the stages of sleep

Sleep fact: The average amount of time it takes to fall asleep is 10 to 20 minutes. If you fall asleep under 5 minutes, then you're probably sleep deprived.

Our internal alarm clocks

Another major driver that regulates our sleep is our circadian rhythm. This is controlled by the suprachiasmatic nucleus

(SCN) basically a biological clock found in the hypothalamus part of the brain. This is the master clock that sets the pace for all other clocks in the body that regulate all bodily processes in a complex series of cogs of activities in all the organs, tissues and cells in the body.

This 'clock' is naturally attuned to daylight and night-time. The SCN can be affected by social activity, temperature, exercise and light which all help regulate the bodily processes.

Light affects our rhythm the most and has a huge impact on our sleep/wake cycle. Light signals to the SCN to keep us alert, whereas darkness induces the production of melatonin, a hormone that induces sleep and helps keep us asleep.

This is why during the winter months, when our bodies see less daylight, we can feel more tired and even depressed. It's also why the blue light in our screens and devices can keep us awake, even in the evenings when we should be winding down.

This finely tuned circadian rhythm can be thrown off balance quite easily. This can be due to a change in routine such as a long-haul flight, anxiety or illness, or even just late-night phone scrolling.

This chaos will cause trouble falling asleep or a disrupted sleep cycle. For example, if we have a 'lie in' at the weekends by Sunday night we struggle to sleep at our usual time because the clock is out of whack.

Sleep apnoea affects this clock too, as the body endures what is essentially a form of regular strangulation at night. Each 'apnoea', is where the breath is held, is essentially the equivalent of someone squeezing your neck tightly. This means our body will have short periods where oxygen stops.

You don't need to be a sleep doctor to understand that's not good for health!

The body keeps the score

We need food and water to survive but however hungry or thirsty we get we cannot force ourselves to eat or drink. However, when we're very tired, our bodies *can* enforce sleep.

This is called a 'microsleep' where we fall asleep for a few seconds, even with eyes open. We could be driving a car or watching TV, or even in a work meeting, but if we are exhausted enough our bodies force tiny naps if we haven't experienced enough NREM or REM in our sleep cycle. This can be a frightening and discombobulating experience but is a clear sign of a sleep disorder of some kind. It's often a sign of sleep apnoea too, although it doesn't happen to everyone. This is one of the reasons driving with untreated severe sleep apnoea is associated with fatal car accidents.

How lack of sleep and sleep apnoea affects all our physiology is explored in depth in Chapter four.

Chapter two

When is snoring a sign of sleep apnoea?

'Laugh and the world laughs with you. Snore and you snore alone.'

Anthony Burgess[7]

Zzzzzz

If you ask anyone to mimic a person who is asleep, they often pretend to snore gently. Snoring can sound peaceful, but it can also be harsh, horn-like, a loud snort, a gasp, often reaching a harsh crescendo before falling silent.

The medical term for snoring is 'stertor', and put simply, it's noisy breathing. And as we get older, things get floppy, so snoring is more likely to become an issue. This is because when we are relaxed our airways naturally relax. The parts of our throat, such as the epiglottis, soft palate and uvula (the dangly bit at the back of the throat), lose their muscle tone and the turbulence of the air passing through makes the noise.

Imagine air whooshing through a tunnel full of flags, but in the body's case, it's flapping pieces of soft cartilage. Once the air hits the back of the throat, it's this that makes the 'snore' sound. An instrument of torture for many co-sleepers to a snorer!

People can snore at any stage of the sleep cycle and apnoea is more common in REM sleep. Snoring can be harmless noisy breathing or be a sign of sleep apnoea but is always an indication of some form of blockage in the airway.

Sleep fact: Human beings began snoring due our evolved bodies which allow us to speak and stand upright. This created changes in our anatomy which causes snoring when asleep. For survival reasons, snoring is not a positive trait in case it alerts predators!

Reasons behind snoring

Everybody snores on occasion. A light rhythmic snore is often a sign of no underlying issues and can be caused by the vibration of soft tissue for numerous reasons.

These include:

1. **Sleep position:** For some people, they only snore when on their back. This is due to the position of the airways blocked by the tongue lolling back due to gravity.
2. **Obstruction of the airways:** This could be congestion of the nasal passages due to a bad cold or rhinitis caused by allergies. An illness causes only a temporary obstruction and snoring might cease once the cold or illness has subsided.

Whereas other obstructions need treating. Snorers can have a deviated septum which means the bone and cartilage between the nose is off centre and can cause breathing issues. Other people have enlarged tonsils or adenoids or polyps.

1. **Alcohol, sleeping tablets or pain killers:** The chemicals in certain drugs or alcohol cause throat and tongue muscles to become relaxed, so they collapse into the airway. Medicating sleep might appear to work short term, but sleep aids should not be used long term, because they don't aid restful REM sleep. Similarly with opioids, especially Fentanyl and Morphine, these painkilling drugs can cause central sleep apnoea (CSA) where the brain doesn't send signals to the body to breathe. This is far less common than obstructive sleep apnoea (OSA),[8] the focus of this book.

2. **Smoking:** Tobacco or vapes can inflame the soft tissue in the throat and airways, creating a smaller passageway.

3. **Body shape and muscle tone:** Poor muscle tone means the airways will close a little bit more. A person's face or jaw shape can also affect snoring. The more recessed your jaw is the smaller the passageways become and the more likely you are to snore. This can be why snoring often runs in families. For example, Asian people quite often have a recessed jaw and despite being slim, develop sleep apnoea.

Likewise, the shape of the soft palate and the uvula affects snoring. If either are particularly long, they can bump and cause the vibration sound, also the tongue could be bulky, have an unusually large base or the mouth could be particularly small. Again, you're not likely to know this unless a sleep specialist investigates.

Sleep fact: In some African cultures the sound of a man snoring is a welcome sign there is a protective man in the house, so fewer African women complain about it!

We don't know for certain how many people snore, but one American study reported that up to 25% of women and around 45% of men do so and snoring is the most common symptom of sleep apnoea, occurring in 75–95% of cases.[9] We also snore at different times in our life. For example, many women snore in later pregnancy or after the menopause. Many men snore in their middle age or after a few drinks. Children can also snore, from birth onwards.

However, the intensity of the snore increases as sleep apnoea becomes more severe. That's why someone with sleep apnoea who snores, often snores very loudly.

What's the difference between the sound of a 'regular snore' and a 'sleep apnoea' snore?

'They say it's not the snoring itself but those anxiety-packed moments in between snorts. It's the waiting for the nasal passages of the person lying beside you to strike again. And strike it always does. In the dark, almost against your will, you produce that special glare reserved for people who cannot control their own behavior.'

Sloane Crosley[10]

You're lying in bed, ear plugs wedged in, next to a partner who is snoring away. But even the ear plugs don't work. You're exhausted, becoming increasingly stressed and wonder how to block out the noise.

A *lawnmower*, a *pig*, a *warthog*, a *coffee machine*, a *stranded whale*, a *buffalo*, *Olympic snoring*, are all descriptions I've heard describing a loved one's snoring caused by sleep apnoea.

Our sleep tests monitor the level of sound, and a sleep apnoea snore can be over 70 decibels. That's the equivalent of a loud washing machine.

A sleep apnoea snore is not a regular constant noise either. It involves gasping and spluttering, guttural wrenches and coughing. Switching off and zoning out the noise of a snore is nigh on impossible; ear plugs or no ear plugs!

Then the noise suddenly stops… Wide awake now, you turn to your sleeping partner, and wait for that next breath to come. This is a common feature of sleep apnoea. Loud, snoring, then a cessation of breath.

The word apnoea is from Greek origin. The word 'a' means 'not' and the word 'pnea' means breathing so together it creates the word: breathless.

There are two types of sleep apnoea. Obstructive sleep apnoea (OSA) (the most common kind), where an obstruction is present, and central sleep apnoea (CSA), where signals in your brain fail to send signals to the muscles to alert the body that you are not getting enough oxygen. Central sleep apnoea affects less than 1% of patients so is far rarer. The common causes of CSA include painkiller usage such as opioids, cardiac issues, and less commonly, brain tumours. Most of what we talk about in this book is obstructive sleep apnoea (OSA).

The loud crescendo of the snore can be followed by snort like gasp. The apnoea is when the air cannot pass. Imagine someone trying to suck through a blocked straw, the straw collapses and in our own airways the tongue sometimes falls back and causes the choking. No wonder the sound of sleep apnoea can be distressing.

This instinctive reflex of gasping ensures a person doesn't stop breathing completely but of course it interrupts the sleep cycle. The more severe the apnoea is, the more interruptions of breath-holding events occur.

This means that the time spent in the REM cycle of sleep gets compressed. Essentially your body won't let you dive into the deep pool of REM sleep because it knows you're drowning during the breath holding.

If this sounds like a horrible night's sleep, it is! Not just for the snorer, but for the person listening to the sound.

Hold on for that breath!

'There is no terror in the bang. Only in the anticipation of it.'

Alfred Hitchcock[11]

Partners of those with sleep apnoea speak of their fearful anticipation, waiting for their loved ones to take the next inhalation of breath. It's anxiety-inducing to watch and for good reason.

Sleep apnoea is measured by AHI which stands for the Apnoea-Hypoapnoea Index. Hypoapnoea means shallow breathing (<50% of a normal breath).

A pause of breath must occur for at least ten seconds for it to count as an apnoea, and we count them over the course of an hour. You add all the apnoeas to the hypo apnoeas over the study and divide by the number of hours. For example, apnoea was 9 per hour and hypo apnoea = 8 per hour the AHI = 8 + 9 =17 per hour.

This determines how severe the sleep apnoea is. Most of these apnoea events will happen in REM stages of the sleep cycle, but they can happen any time.

- Mild sleep apnoea is between 5 and 15 events per hour.
- Moderate sleep apnoea is between 15 and 30 events per hour.
- Severe sleep apnoea is 30 or more events per hour.

So, this means for someone with severe sleep apnoea they stop breathing over 240 times over the course of an average 8-hour sleep. Sometimes people stop breathing for up to a minute at a time.

It's not just the number of times you stop breathing but also how profoundly low your oxygen levels drop to.

That's 240 times your body is experiencing the equivalent of strangulation each night, every night and your oxygen levels could plummet to 50% or below triggering cardiac events such as a heart attack. No wonder sleep apnoea knocks off a few brain cells and triggers heart attacks and strokes.

Other signs that indicate sleep apnoea includes needing the bathroom multiple times at night, waking with a headache and/or a sore throat and experiencing excessive daytime sleepiness. It can also happen that sleep apnoea begins mildly then progresses to become moderate then severe.

Children can develop sleep apnoea too. We examine this in detail in Chapter seven. Children with sleep apnoea have poor concentration spans at school or disruptive behaviour, due to the disrupted sleep cycle and exhaustion.

What makes you more likely to have sleep apnoea?

There are several factors that make us more likely to have sleep apnoea.

Genetics: If your father or mother snored and had sleep apnoea (almost certainly it won't have been diagnosed as the science of sleep apnoea is so new), then be wary of inheriting this condition yourself. This can be due to the physical traits, such as a small, recessed jaw, or propensity for putting on weight.

Obesity: The bigger your BMI, the more likely you are to have sleep apnoea, the correlation is linear.[12] This is due to the narrowing of the upper airway due to the excess fat. People who are obese, that's having a BMI of over 30, have twice as many sleep problems as those with low BMIs. If you lose excess weight, it is possible to cure yourself of sleep apnoea.

To calculate your BMI, take your weight in kilogrammes, divide it by your height squared. For example, your weight is 70kg and you are 1.73m tall, the calculation will be 70 ÷ 1.73 × 1.73 = 23.41.

Your BMI should be below 30, ideally between 18.5 and 24.9.

Big neck: The size of the neck is also a criterion. The wider your neck, the more likely it is to develop sleep apnoea. Very muscular athletes can have this issue too. The average rugby player or overweight lorry driver is frequently seen in my clinics.

Gender: Around 8% of men have sleep apnoea compared to around 6% of women. Women are more likely to develop sleep apnoea after the menopause (it doubles!), especially if they are not on HRT. The bulk of my patients are overweight, middle-aged men who have been struggling to sleep for years. But that doesn't mean sleep apnoea doesn't affect slim men or women and of course children too. Basically, anyone is at risk of having sleep apnoea or developing it. That's why we should all be aware of it.

BAME backgrounds: Research into patients from Black, Asian and minority ethnic backgrounds are notoriously poorly studied. However, research does suggest that those from a BAME backgrounds are more likely to have sleep apnoea.

In one American study, Black people presented with OSA at a younger age than their white counterparts.[13] In addition, another study found that Black (Afro-Caribbean) people over the age of 65 were 2.5 times more likely than white people to

have severe OSA.[14] This is very similar to the development
of hypertension in this group and OSA may very well be
the cause. Note that this group tend to have relatively large
tongues, and this could be the anatomical trigger for OSA.

Pregnant women: Towards the third trimester around a third
of women report snoring and sleep apnoea can be developed.
Among obese pregnant women the figure is around 15–20%
develop sleep apnoea.[15]

Postmenopausal women: There are few studies in the UK
on this, but in the US, a study has shown that between 47%
and 67% of postmenopausal women develop sleep apnoea.[16]
The US has a bigger obesity issue than the UK, so this could
be a factor in the higher number, although we're only about
five to ten years behind our friends across the pond. Another
European study, however, has noted that females now
represent up to 40–50% of patients in all sleep clinics.[17]

Children with big tonsils: Around 3% of the paediatric
population has sleep apnoea, but almost all of it goes
undiagnosed. A child with large tonsils and adenoids is a big
indicating factor for sleep apnoea.

The *only* way to find out if your snoring is dangerous
– because it's sleep apnoea related – or if it's harmless is by
doing a professional sleep study and get diagnosed by a sleep
specialist. There is no other way of finding out.

If you're reading this book and want to know immediately
if it's likely that you, your partner or your child has sleep
apnoea, then turn to page 48 to fill out the questionnaire.

Chapter three

Why sleep apnoea kills

'OSA is *The Lord of the Rings* – it binds all other conditions together.'

Michael Oko

Sleep apnoea is a killer because it affects so many of our body's systems as they all require oxygen to function. Each apnoea means you stop breathing and oxygen levels can dip below 90% and go down to 50% or lower, way lower than the 95–99% range the body needs. The more apnoea episodes a person has and the more profound the oxygen desaturation, the less oxygen their vital organs are getting.

Every time the breath is held, the body automatically goes into a 'fight' or 'flight' response, as triggered by the autonomic nervous system (ANS) because the body is in panic mode, in need of oxygen. The ANS is responsible for all the automatic reflexes in our bodies, such as heart rate, digestion and certain reflexes like vomiting, urination, coughing, sneezing and swallowing.

The fight or flight system means adrenaline is poured into the blood stream and cortisol levels shoot up, which triggers the heart to respond by increasing your heart rate and blood pressure. It also inhibits insulin activity as you need the high glucose to 'flee the stressful event'.

If each apnoea is the equivalent of someone squeezing your neck each time for at least 10 seconds, it's no surprise it's not a good thing! But let's do a deep dive of exactly what parts of our body and minds sleep apnoea affects.

Reading this will make it clear why everyone with sleep apnoea needs to get help.

Head

Each breath-holding event causes the body's fight or flight system to react as if it is about to be attacked by a bear. The ANS system, however, cannot keep your airway open at this time, so that's why people wake up with a bolt sometimes, or gasp for air.

During this event some patients report having vivid dreams, of near drowning or someone chasing them. Some feel literally in fear of their life because the brain is essentially screaming the signal to '*Wake up! Start breathing again!*'. The fright in your dream is a fright to wake up, as if being chased by a bear is happening in real time.

The heart races and sometimes patients wake up with a sense of '*That was a close one!*'. The response to the heart racing increases the blood pressure and this causes a tendency for the blood to clot.

If a patient has severe sleep apnoea (that's 30 breath holds in an hour or more) and is left untreated it can have a catastrophic detrimental effect.

One study revealed – over a 12-year period – nearly a third of patients with untreated severe sleep apnoea *will* have a stroke. Around 15% will die of a cardiac arrest in that time period.[18]

This is because the stress caused by adrenaline also causes the blood platelets to become super adhesive and can form clots very quickly. These things tend to happen at night too.

Sleep fact: When you sleep deeply, blood pressure lowers and heart rate reduces by about 10–15%, giving the heart a much-needed rest too as the heart only 'breathes' or gets oxygenated when it is not contracting i.e., between beats.

Mood

Excessive tiredness has a direct impact on our mood and cognitive decision making. We are more likely to suffer from irritability, anxiety, depression and feel out of control. Mood swings throw up challenges when faced with work and family responsibilities.

When overtired, our ability to emotionally regulate is diminished making it harder to make decisions, judgments and keep our cool. As a result, relationships with loved ones and family all suffer.

Daytime exhaustion

Tired people suffer from brain fog, concentration lapses, difficulty with ordinary tasks. Studies reveal work productivity can slump by 30%.

Tired people are also dangerous. Especially if they're driving or in charge of machinery. It's estimated approximately

20% of all fatal traffic accidents that happen are caused by people who are suffering from fatigue. We explore the cost of this in Chapter nine. Sleep apnoea not only kills the patient but sometimes other people.

Cardiovascular system

Heart

The breath-holding events – the apnoeas – affect the heart badly. Acute stress, the fight or flight response, makes your heart sensitized by the adrenaline, so it beats harder and faster. If the heart pumps against resistance and the process of the blood coming in and out isn't in sync anymore it's quite catastrophic. This is because only when the heart is in between beats does it receive the necessary oxygen.

If you sleep deeply through the night your heart rate drops from about 72 to 62 beats per minute. So, over an 8-hour night that is 4,800 fewer beats and more time for the heart to rest. With apnoea the heart rate can exceed 120 during the apnoea due to the release of adrenaline. Atrial fibrillation (rapid and irregular heartbeats) is associated with this increased release of adrenaline which in turn is associated with an increased risk of stroke, dementia and heart failure.

I have seen patients with atrial fibrillation revert to normal sinus rhythm when on CPAP therapy, avoiding the need for cardioversion (shocking the heart back into a normal rhythm). Indeed, if they keep needing cardioversions then undiagnosed OSA should be considered.

This is why the risk of having a heart attack or stroke tends to be heightened at nighttime – between 3am and 4am – and also associated with increased cortisol levels.

Hypertension: Obstructive sleep apnoea is a leading cause of high blood pressure. This has a direct impact on the heart because it must work so much harder against higher resistance from the arterial walls caused but the increased tone, due to excessive adrenaline release. Normal blood pressure should be around 120/80 where the 120 is the systolic (when the heart has contracted and pushed blood into the arteries – a bit like blowing up a balloon) and the 80 is the diastolic pressure (when the resting tone in the arteries is at its lowest – or the balloon has deflated partially). In fit and healthy people their resting heart rate will be low, say 60–100 beats per minutes. For a super fit person, a trained sportsperson, for example, then 40 beats per minutes is possible. The lower the heart rate the better, but for people with sleep apnoea, their heart will skyrocket, every night.

High blood pressure damages the arteries, making them less elastic and in turns this decreases the blood flowing to the heart. This increases the risk of heart disease.

Cardiac arrythmia: With sleep apnoea you are four times more likely to have atrial fibrillation again triggered by high adrenaline levels released by apnoea (where the hearts upper chambers don't beat regularly). This increases the risk of damage to the heart, blood clots and strokes. Some people feel their heart pumping wildly, but others don't have any sensation at all.

Congestive heart failure: This is when the heart has started to fail as a pump and fluids build up in the legs and lungs. Even with moderate OSA there is an increased mortality rate.

Stroke: Sufferers with moderate to severe OSA are three times as likely to suffer a stroke. The worse the sleep apnoea is, the more likely they are to have a stroke. Researchers have found stroke patients often suffer from OSA but do not know about it, this is because there is so little awareness.

Body weight

What comes first… the sleep apnoea or the weight gain? It's a chicken and egg scenario. Often, people with sleep apnoea are battling tiredness during the day and so reach for food. This is because tiredness causes the hormone ghrelin to increase which increases appetite and decreases the hormone leptin which makes a person feel full up.

Tiredness also affects our cognitive abilities, to think clearly and make positive decisions. When our decision-making processes get compromised with tiredness, people think: '*Sod it, I want the cake!*' and our ability to reason with ourselves to make healthier choices goes out the window.

This is also the result of having experienced a stress event in the night, so our bodies look for food in the morning. This is like a bear trying to tuck in a fat juicy salmon, in preparation to enter hibernation for a winter that never comes. It's comfort food but also a reaction to our hormones.

And where does this excess weight and fat go on the body? The heart, abdomen and around the soft tissues too, which includes the neck and airways. This affects our breathing by narrowing our airways with extra padding of fat when we sleep, and apnoea is more likely to be a problem.

We are in an obesity crisis in the UK. More than one in four adults are now obese in the UK and this figure is rising steeply. This means more people than ever will be suffering from sleep apnoea in the future. Thus, we will see more dementia and diabetes too.

Kidneys/bladder

Sleep apnoea causes the need to wee a lot at night. This is because the release of adrenaline causes blood pressure to rocket, which increases profusion to the kidneys which in turn produces more urine. If your bladder is full up, then your brain will wake up your body to release it.

This can happen multiple times a night to people with sleep apnoea and is called Nocturia. I've had patients who need to get up and wee as much as six or seven times a night. Exhausting!

Sex drive

When I meet a reluctant male patient in my clinic, I often tell him straight: 'You soon won't be able to get your pecker up!'. The lack of oxygen causes tiredness and results in lower levels of testosterone. This has a knock-on effect on much of a man's body. His sex drive will take a dip, and he will struggle to get and maintain an erection. Other side effects include loss of muscle tone, hair and even body height and bone strength. Low levels of this hormone can also affect a man's mood. Untreated sleep apnoea causes impotence.

If I ever meet a patient who has little or no interest in sex, it's one of the clearest signs that they are not a well person. It's unsurprising that patients do not feel in the mood when they are just so exhausted.

Pain relief

Some pain-relieving medications can cause sleep apnoea. For example, if you've got a bad back and prescribed Fentanyl patches, this is likely to affect your sleep. All the opiates have a similar impact, interfering with messages from the brain and signalling, and is something to monitor if they're prescribed.

Drugs need to be reviewed regularly to understand the impact on the body. Every person on medication needs to be knowledgeable about their own medications and the way it interacts in the body to understand the full impact, because everyone's reaction is individual.

It's important to understand that many patients present with multiple health problems – each of which is another additional burden. About 38% of my patients have disabilities or other health issues.

Gastro reflux

During the apnoea episodes, your diaphragm pulls down, the chest expands, trying to help suck in air that does not enter. This negative pressure leads to sucking up the contents of the stomach, to the back of the throat. Acid lands in the throat, and if this happens repeatedly at night, it means waking up with a sore throat.

About 60% of OSA patients experience this and sometimes if it happens at night, it can be extremely distressing. Patients report having to sit bolt upright as the acid hits the larynx as this goes into spasm to stop acid getting to the lungs.

They then must wait until the larynx relaxes before getting air in or out. Some patients describe having to sit calmly on the side of the bed for a few seconds (this can feel like ages!).

More commonly patients will be aware of 'something at the back of my throat' and will keep clearing the throat of mucus that builds up as a result of contact with acid. The constant clearing of the throat and sometimes huskiness causes the patient to be anxious and become overly aware of sensations at the back of the throat.

Treatment includes lifestyle changes such as avoiding trigger foods – e.g., pepper, spicy food and alcohol. Avoid eating late (allow 4–6 hours for your food to digest – so eat at 6pm if bedtime is about 10pm). Try drugs that reduce acid production such as Omeprazole, Lansoprazole, etc.

Immune system

Sleep apnoea compromises the immune system because you're not getting the restorative sleep you need. Studies have shown if you have a vaccination during a period where you're not sleeping well, it will be less effective.[19]

Tiredness means you're more suspectable to other infections too, like colds and flu. One study also shows untreated sleep apnoea is linked to a higher chance of being hospitalized with influenza, for example.[20]

Another study revealed that people who sleep for 7 hours regularly were as much as 300% less likely to get an infection.[21] This is because during deep sleep immune systems kick into action. The job of white blood cells is to identify pathogens, attack and remove them.

During this process, the white blood cells release a protein called cytokines which signals to other white blood cells to prepare for attack. When asleep our bodies slow down and this gives more energy towards this process, so it works more effectively.

Real world implications for timing of drug delivery at night

'A "robust" Spanish study of more than 19,000 patients found that taking the medication so that it works overnight cuts the risk of heart-related death and disease nearly in half. The same medication ingested at different times of the day actually has different pharmacological properties, behaving like totally different medications,' said the study's lead author, Ramon Hermida, director of the Bioengineering and Chrono-biology Labs at the University of Vigo in Spain.

- Short-acting statins: more effective as we produce more cholesterol at night.
- Long-acting insulin: evening or bedtime to provide better insulin control.

- PPI's: Nexium, etc., 1–2 hours before an evening meal, ideally 4–6 hour before bedtime for maximum benefit.

Diseases

This section highlights the most common chronic illnesses which OSA can cause or is associated with.

Diabetes

Type two diabetes is associated with weight gain. With an obesity crisis gripping the UK and Europe, already there are about five million people in the UK alone with diabetes and this figure is set to rise and is said to consume 10% of the NHS budget already. Incredibly, sleep apnoea is as common as diabetes, yet nobody is talking about it!

Diabetes is a metabolic disease which causes blood sugar levels to become too high which leads to heart attacks, strokes, kidney disease, nerve damage and eye and foot issues.

Controlling insulin levels (which lowers blood glucose) is almost impossible unless the apnoea is controlled. This is because once you're in fight or flight, adrenaline needs glucose to burn. Plus, your body believes it's running from the bear remember!

Adrenaline is the king of the hormones in the sense that it uses up so much energy, it is the chief. Insulin is needed to control the blood sugar levels, therefore it becomes a terribly complex seesaw, trying to balance both, especially if you have sleep apnoea.

What comes first? The development of sleep apnoea (which causes excess hunger that leads to obesity) or obesity that leads to sleep apnoea? We simply don't have enough research to know.

If you have sleep apnoea, however, you are more likely to gain weight and become diabetic.

Cancer

A recent meta-analysis with over 32 million patients has shown that people with OSA are 1.5 times more likely to get cancer. Individuals with OSA are more likely to develop tumours, and the incidence is related to the severity of OSA.

A telomere is compound structure at the end of a chromosome. As we age, they get shorter leading to inactive cells eventually. We are yet to fully understand this relationship, but it is known that leukocyte telomere length (LTL) is shortened in OSA patients and shortening of telomere length correlated with increasing age, and the apnoea-hypopnea index (AHI). Telomere length is important as it helps us to reproduce cells with accuracy, but it naturally gets shorter over time.

Telomerase is crucial – think of it as the immortality enzyme – in the processes of a lot of chronic conditions and one of the reasons you can get cancer is if the cells are not perfectly reproduced each time. Instead, abnormal and defective cells are made.

Being obese raises the risk of developing breast cancer, both before and after the menopause.[22] Being obese also affects cancer treatment with chemotherapy being less effective for obese women.

A meta-analysis study revealed that the 5-year breast cancer survival rate for obese or overweight women was 55.6%, whereas it was 79.9% for women with normal weight.[23]

I am currently working with NHS breast cancer patients to offer sleep apnoea treatment to improve the treatment outcomes of patients.

Potential implications for cancer?

- Thousands of rhythmically expressed genes metabolize, transport or are the targets of drugs. For drugs with rapid pharmacokinetics (the absorption, distribution, metabolism and excretion of drugs), circadian time could influence efficacy and/or toxicity and thus their therapeutic index.[24]

- Chemotherapy over night? 'Timing is everything, and here we have molecular data showing why this is especially true with regard to cancer', Dr Sancar said. 'By hitting cancer cells with chemotherapy at a time when their ability to repair themselves is minimal, you should be able to maximize effectiveness and minimize side effects of treatment.'[25] In mice, levels of one DNA damage repair protein called xeroderma pigmentosa A (XPA) repaired damaged DNA samples 6–7 times faster at night!

- Radiotherapy in the evenings? Could this be more effective for the same dose?

- Ensuring all sleep issues are addressed before starting therapy to maximize benefit?

Dementia

Dementia is the term for declining brain function and the most common kind of dementia is Alzheimer's disease.

One in 11 people in the UK over the age of 65 have dementia in some form. It's estimated by 2030 the number of people with dementia will be over a million. We are essentially sleepwalking into a dementia tsunami especially as we lack the social services needed to deal with the high needs of these patients.

Sleep apnoea may be the missing link (it's a hypothesis and the leap to a scientific fact is a very high bar to achieve and prove causality) between high blood pressure and Alzheimer's disease as previously mentioned. The glymphatic system in stage 3 or deep sleep clears out toxins but sleep apnoea stops this from happening efficiently as you are kept in light sleep for a disproportionate amount of time. Sleep apnoea also raises blood pressure, which makes it harder for blood to pump and the glymphatic system to function effectively too.

It's estimated that 40% of people with dementia have sleep apnoea, but most of them are undiagnosed.

An interesting group to look at are Down syndrome patients. Many of whom suffer with OSA and early onset Alzheimer's disease with around 50% of patients presenting symptoms in their 60s. These patients can do well with CPAP if they wish to use it. Many are not brought to sleep clinics due to lack of awareness or the assumption that they will not tolerate the use of a mask.

At the very least, lack of sleep affects our memories, our ability to learn, our short-term thinking and cognitive function.

This chapter has been a stark explanation of why sleep apnoea is known as the (not-so-) silent killer. That's the bad news.

The good news is, there are very effective sleep apnoea therapies available that can reduce all of the above side effects, increasing the chances of a long and healthy life.

So, if sleep apnoea can be cured, what are you waiting for?

.

Chapter four

Have you or your partner got sleep apnoea? Find out!

The only way to get sleep apnoea diagnosed is to get a sleep test done by a professional sleep clinic. How to navigate the easiest pathway to the clinic, especially for a reluctant partner who snores, is examined in detail later in the book.

But before even making a GP appointment for a referral I recommend filling out the two questionnaires in this chapter. If a person's snoring is relatively harmless, they will score between 1 and 3. If a person should have a referral for sleep apnoea, they'll score over 3 and if they score over 6, the chances are, they have severe sleep apnoea.

The first questionnaire is called *Stop Bang*. The specific questions were developed by an American anaesthetist, Dr Chung, who wanted a rapid questionnaire to ask his patients to assess their suitability before he put them under anaesthetic.

If a patient has undiagnosed sleep apnoea and is put to sleep for an operation this can be life threatening because breathing must be carefully monitored at this time.

It is extremely important to know if a patient has OSA before any operation. These are the four key stages as to why:

- **Intubation:** OSA patients can be very difficult to intubate, so this is usually undertaken by the most senior anaesthetist.
- **Maintain general anaesthetic safely:** It's best to try and make any medical procedure as short as possible by having the senior surgeon do the case and avoid opiate analgesia.
- **Immediate post operative:** Very close monitoring in the recovery room must happen. For example, patients must be placed on CPAP that they should have brought in with them (you should be told to bring this into the hospital at pre-assessment appointment).
- **Overnight stay:** Most OSA patients are not suitable for day case procedures and any operations should not be undertaken in hospitals that do not have high dependency or intensive care beds.

This questionnaire is a really easy way to work out if the signs of sleep apnoea are evident which is important.

The second questionnaire is called the *Epworth Sleepiness Scale* (ESS). In terms of sleep medicine, 'sleepiness' means 'the probability, ease or speed of making the transition from alert wakefulness, through drowsiness, to sleep under a given set of circumstances.'[26]

Dr Murray Johns developed the ESS for adults in the 1990s to assess the 'daytime sleepiness' of patients in his private sleep clinic. It's named after Epworth Hospital in Melbourne, Australia, where Murray established the Epworth Sleep Centre in 1988.

The ESS is a questionnaire with eight simple questions on a 4-point scale (0–3), asking patients to rate their usual chances of nodding off or falling sound asleep while engaged in eight different activities such as driving.

The higher the ESS score, the higher that person's average sleep propensity in daily life or their 'daytime sleepiness'. It takes no more than a few minutes to answer and is available in many different languages.

The disadvantage to using this scale is that a person who has depression could score highly and this should be factored in.

Either of these questionnaires can be done by a partner or the person who snores. They can be very revelatory!

How can sleep apnoea be dealt with? Quickly and easily, is the answer. Skip to Chapter ten if you'd like to find out what pathways I recommend and what treatments are available.

But meanwhile we explore why men and women treat snoring and sleep apnoea differently and why our culture doesn't take sleep seriously.

The Stop Bang questionnaire

Is it possible that you have obstructive sleep apnoea (OSA)?

Please answer the following questions below to determine if you might be at risk.

Snoring?
Do you snore loudly (loud enough to be heard through closed doors or your bed-partner elbows you for snoring at night)?

Yes ☐ No ☐

Tired?
Do you often feel tired, fatigued or sleepy during the daytime (such as falling asleep during driving or talking to someone)?

Yes ☐ No ☐

Observed?
Has anyone observed you stop breathing or choking/gasping during your sleep?

Yes ☐ No ☐

Pressure?
Do you have or are you being treated for high blood pressure?

Yes ☐ No ☐

Body mass index (BMI) more than 35kg/m²?

Body mass index calculator = weight (kg) ÷ height² (metres squared)

Height:

Weight:

BMI:

Yes ☐ No ☐

Age older than 50?

Yes ☐ No ☐

Neck size large? (Measured around Adam's apple)

Is your shirt collar 16 inches / 40cm or larger?

Yes ☐ No ☐

Gender

Male?

Yes ☐ No ☐

For general population

OSA – Low risk: Yes to 0–3 questions

OSA – Intermediate risk: Yes to 4–5 questions

OSA – High risk: Yes to 6–8 questions

Source: Property of University Health Network. Modified from: Chung, F. et al. (2008) *Anesthesiology*, 108: 812–821; Chung, F. et al. (2012) *British Journal of Anaesthesia*, 108: 768–775; Chung, F. et al. (2014) *Journal of Clinical Sleep Medicine*, Sept 2014.

The Epworth questionnaire

Situation/chance of dozing

Sitting and reading

| Would never doze | Slight chance of dozing | Moderate chance of dozing | High chance of dozing |

Watching TV

| Would never doze | Slight chance of dozing | Moderate chance of dozing | High chance of dozing |

Sitting, inactive in a public place (e.g., a theatre or a meeting)

| Would never doze | Slight chance of dozing | Moderate chance of dozing | High chance of dozing |

As a passenger in a car for an hour without a break

| Would never doze | Slight chance of dozing | Moderate chance of dozing | High chance of dozing |

Lying down to rest in the afternoon when circumstances permit

| Would never doze | Slight chance of dozing | Moderate chance of dozing | High chance of dozing |

Sitting and talking to someone

| *Would never doze* | *Slight chance of dozing* | *Moderate chance of dozing* | *High chance of dozing* |

Sitting quietly after lunch without alcohol

| *Would never doze* | *Slight chance of dozing* | *Moderate chance of dozing* | *High chance of dozing* |

In a car, while stopped for a few minutes in traffic

| *Would never doze* | *Slight chance of dozing* | *Moderate chance of dozing* | *High chance of dozing* |

Part two

Snore wars!

Chapter five

A man's world

'Michael Oko is the only consultant I have ever met who has grasped that women are often the guardians of men's health.'

Isabel, wife of a current patient

A round 60% of my patients are men. Many of them are overweight, middle management types who have been ordered by their wives to get help for their snoring. When they arrive at the clinic, most of them don't want to be there.

From my 18 years clinical experience as a consultant, men and women deal with sleep issues very differently. This sounds like a sexist generalization (and there are always exceptions to the rule!), but most men I meet, initially don't want help for their snoring and are in denial of health consequences. Many of our sleep specialist nurses agree. As one of my sleep clinic nurses says: 'Everyone who comes to our clinic is always on their knees, either man or woman. But it's the men who always need more of a push to come in the first place.'

That's because, as a rule, men are rubbish at looking after themselves. On average women outlive men by five or six years as they're more likely to seek medical help and in my view, are far more pragmatic and take less risks. Studies back this up. A National Health Interview survey in 2014, revealed that men are 50% less likely than women to go and see their GP for a health issue.[27]

Whereas a National Pharmacy Association study concluded that nine out of ten men wouldn't go to a doctor or pharmacy unless their condition was serious.[28] For every six visits women make to the doctor, men only make four. Many never go at all.

That is why single men tend to die younger. They also do not have a partner to tell them to go and get help.

This is a big problem when it comes to sleep apnoea because more men than women suffer from it and so are more likely to die from it. But they are less likely to seek help!

Add to this mix, sleep apnoea is not on the radar of all GPs so it means even getting a referral can feel like a battle.

Of course, our cultural approach towards sleep and snoring does not help. Snoring is seen as annoying but there's little understanding about its dangerous underlying causes. Partly because we don't value sleep as a society so don't make restorative sleep a priority. Most of us, man, or woman, accept tiredness as part of modern life and change the subject.

By the time patients arrive in our waiting room, they will have struggled for long sleepless years. They'll either have self-medicated or been multiple times to see a GP and received inappropriate help. While others will have tried useless snoring remedies.

The relationship battlelines

'You can see me – the sleep specialist – or the divorce lawyers, it's your choice, chief.'

Dr Michael Oko to a male patient

Snoring is often cited on divorce papers under 'unreasonable behaviour'. Most divorces are also initiated by women and not men. Gavin Rossdale once quoted: 'Happy wife is a happy life' and that is never truer when it comes to snoring.

I have seen first-hand how years of tolerating sleep disturbance can turn love to hate. Sometimes the tension between couples is so palpable in the clinic I feel like a hostage negotiator.

There is little official data on the impact of snoring on relationships, but anecdotally, sleep specialists and charity groups, like Relate, acknowledge the devastation.

Specsavers were promoting earplugs recently and did a survey of 2,000 people, which found that nearly one in ten considered splitting up from their partner due to snoring. According to their data, the average person can lose up to 68 minutes of sleep per night, to the sound of a partner snoring and that 28% were woken every night by it.[29]

Among the snorers, apparently, over 40% said they felt guilty about their snoring but around a quarter admitted they were not bothered at all!

I've heard husbands say: 'Sod it, it's not my problem!' because they cannot hear themselves snore. But for their wives it's often a line in the sand, and the exhaustion alongside the defensiveness leads to divorces.

I've had couples who barely sat down in the waiting room when the man stormed out, not wanting to engage with a doctor about his snoring. I've met couples on the brink of divorce, only saved by a sleep apnoea diagnosis and treatment. Others who have wives who have withheld sex or banished their partner to the spare room until they've got help.

All couples I meet are tired, fed up and desperately want life to get better. Which is the easy bit because therapy for sleep apnoea is available quickly and easily and can literally turn a life around within 72 hours. CPAP machines or other treatments stop snoring when nothing else works.

All hope is not lost, even if a relationship feels mortally wounded.

A macho world

'There ain't no way to find out why a snorer can't hear himself snore.'

Mark Twain[30]

Many men don't like medical intervention because of the macho culture we exist in. The default setting for most males is: 'Unless my leg is falling off, I'll stick a plaster on it' or 'Unless I am about to die, then what's the point in worrying?'

I've met male patients who are seriously more concerned about being incapacitated than actual death! One of them said they couldn't stand being left disabled, but if he was dead, well… he wouldn't know about it. The comedian Micky Flanagan articulates this well in his stand-up routine, where he tells of a conversation with his wife about her fears around economic security if he had a stroke.[31] In a very funny exchange, Micky says the idea of him being incapacitated after a stroke and watching his wife turn up to visit him in a care home with a new handbag is what bothers him the most.

With varying attitudes towards preventative medicine, explaining the dangers of sleep apnoea can be challenging.

Many men simply don't want to know, unless it's urgent. Instead of seeking help for snoring, many men get annoyed at their partners for complaining about something that seems so common.

Often, men view the potential sleep apnoea therapy to be emasculating. The gold standard therapy for severe and moderate sleep apnoea is the CPAP machine, a clever device that pumps pressurized air into the mouth or nose. We explore this miracle machine in Chapter eleven.

However, many men don't like the idea of wearing a mask and a sleep treatment turning them into a 'patient'. Other younger men say they'd die of embarrassment at the idea of slipping on a sleep mask after bringing back a young lady, for example.

I often tell male patients to think of the CPAP mask as some kind of movie prop. I tell them to think of *Top Gun*, *Bandits at 12 O'clock* or Darth Vader's mask. The force is strong with this one!

These jokes at least raise a smile during what can be a challenging conversation. Although, women find this less funny and prefer a more sensitive approach. But before we get there, how do we persuade men to attend a sleep clinic in the first place?

Pick the battles in order to win the war

In many homes there is a snoring battle happening, and our clinic is often the final frontier. But how do you encourage your partner (especially male partners!), to make the appointment in the first place?

Partners have leverage on their other halves, everyone knows this. I don't advocate manipulation, but when it comes to getting someone tested for sleep apnoea sometimes a little bit of clever persuasion helps.

Recognizing what buttons to press and when to press them can be the start of successful skirmishes before picking the fight to get that all important sleep study done. But let's break this down:

- Step one is encouraging the partner to accept there is a problem.
- Step two is getting them to see a GP.
- Step three is the sleep study.
- Step four is getting a confirmed diagnosis.
- Step five is embracing the appropriate therapy and using it.

But first we need a ceasefire. Chances are both partners are tired and angry with each other. They need to stop swiping before a calm discussion can take place.

Often the snoring partner can immediately be on the defensive taking up rear guard action during step one, which is the identification of a problem.

So, first of all, read this book from cover to cover. Arm yourself with information. Sleep apnoea and why loud snoring is a symptom is a completely new subject for the majority of people.

Then the first step could be a conversation that starts like this: 'Darling, neither of us are sleeping well, and I am worried about your health. How about we make an appointment to see a GP? I can come and support you?'

If that fails, retreat and regroup. Maybe you need to enlist other family members or sympathetic friends to have a word? Next step could be to gently begin sharing facts on sleep apnoea and suggest doing the *Stop Bang* questionnaire in Chapter four together.

If your partner still refuses, perhaps do the questionnaire on their behalf, and then show them the results when they're in a better mood.

Relationship counsellor, Wendy Gregory,[32] gave me these three valuable top tips when approaching a no-go health topic.

- Don't try to goad or nag the person into taking action. Choose a time to talk when both of you are in a calm and peaceful mood.
- Be sure what you want to say and say it clearly once, e.g., facts, statistics, etc. The more you try to persuade someone who doesn't want to do something the less likely they are to do it.
- Say what you want and then say: 'I really think it would be a good idea to see the GP, but of course, it is up to you.' You are then handing the responsibility over to them and allowing them to think it was their idea!

Another idea, which I've heard has been effective, is to download an app for the phone which monitors snoring levels, such as SnoreLab or Sleep Cycle.

The app will pick up how 'loud' the snorer is and in the morning the person can see how and when they snored the previous night. This has been a major wake up call for many male patients who were in complete denial about the extent of their problem. The app shows data which can't be argued with.

One client I know drove his poor wife mad with his loud snoring for almost a decade before he used the SnoreLab app. The next morning, he looked at the app data and realized his snore registered as 'epic' – the loudest volume the device could pick up. Suddenly he fully appreciated how loud he was at night and instead of simply saying: 'I can't help it!' he apologized to his wife for the first time.

Bedroom divorce

Many of the older couples I meet, sleep apart. I call this 'bedroom divorce'. Often, they are in their 50s, the children have flown the nest, and they have a spare room in the house. Sex has fallen down the agenda and so sleeping apart is not an issue.

This works out okay for some couples but is not for everyone. Many married couples want to share a bedroom, but loud snoring makes it unbearable.

Wendy Gregory agrees that snoring is a big bone of contention between men and women because it ultimately affects intimacy too.

She says:

'Snoring almost always impacts on a relationship, as would anything that causes sleep disturbance. A partner can feel resentful, but it can also impact massively on the intimacy in a relationship.

When we're exhausted, we don't generally feel receptive to our partner's sexual advances. In many cases the woman resorts to sleeping in a different bedroom, which in turn leads to her partner feeling rejected sexually.'

On top of this, men who have sleep apnoea often suffer from impotence, and this causes further feelings of emasculation.

Grinding down the defences

When they're in the defensive position, men often use the following arguments to avoid help for snoring and sleep apnoea. Here are some common statements made by male patients with my replies in italics below.

1. **'Snoring can't be stopped, I have tried nose strips, pillows, <insert any other faddy anti-snoring products>'**
   Yes, it can. Most over the counter therapies for snoring don't work. You haven't tried the gold standard NICE recommended therapy which is a CPAP machine. It comes with over 30 different masks and there is something almost everyone feels comfortable with. If not, we can look at other clinically proven therapies. I have an 80% success rate with patients trying therapies.

2. **'Snoring is not a big deal, most men do it'**
   It is a big deal if it's sleep apnoea. Long term serious health issues are almost guaranteed and you're more likely to feel exhausted, depressed and be overweight. Worst case scenarios are you will become impotent or drop dead.

3. **'I don't want to waste a doctor's time'**

   You'll be wasting much more of a doctor's time if you get sick from all the illnesses associated with sleep apnoea. Sleep apnoea is my specialism, this is what I am here for.

4. **'I don't have time to take off work for this'**

   You will end up taking more time off work with the sleep apnoea linked illness. Prevention is always better than a cure and you can prevent this. Plus, workdays will feel far easier if you're not exhausted. Patients report feeling more productive at work and definitely feeling more energetic and positive. It's time very well spent.

5. **'I am scared in case they find something wrong' (they're unlikely to verbalize this aloud)**

   There are effective treatments, cures even. Sleep apnoea is one of the easiest sleep disorders to treat and if you don't like the initial therapy, we can try something else to find what works.

6. **'If I find out I have obstructive sleep apnoea it could affect my driver's license, can't it?'**

   All sleep apnoea patients can carry on driving cars, taxis, lorries, coaches and even planes if they want to. We can help with the DVLA compliance needed, and it shouldn't stop you from getting treated.

7. **'I am not using a CPAP machine so there is no point'**

   If you are really against using a CPAP machine, we can discuss other options. There is a mandibular device that sits in the mouth like a rugby guard, or we can look at surgery.

Many of my reluctant patients on CPAP fall in love their machine, don't knock it until you try it!

In extreme cases, when male patients say point blank, they do not want a sleep study, I explain the brutal statistics behind untreated sleep apnoea. I explain to them what they can expect over the next 12 years.

Over a 12-year period, people who suffer from untreated severe sleep apnoea have a 30% higher chance of a stroke and a 15% chance of a sudden cardiac arrest. It's as stark as that.

I always urge my patients to get themselves checked, don't mess about. But if they still refuse, I can't force them.

It's then I suggest they go away and think about it.

Minimizing collateral damage

If my male patient has children, I will also mention the positive knock-on effects of therapy on their ability to parent. When the adults in a house are exhausted, everyone suffers, including the children. So many of my patients report they do not have any energy left by the end of the day and at weekends for anything else, including spending time with their families.

Many try and nap at weekends to make up for sleep, or simply feel too low to take an interest in what their family is doing.

That's not even mentioning the chances of ill health being significantly higher. Who wants to see their children live into adulthood and meet their grandchildren? Everyone does.

I often gently explain to my patients who are reluctant to listen that any treatment benefits the whole family. They will have more energy for their children, be more patient, feel more like spending quality time with them. They will stop being grumpy and irritable and start enjoying life again. They are more likely to live longer, healthier lives.

Few people can argue with that. Even if they do, I never ever give up on patients, even those who are annoyed and don't want to know. I've had male patients who have refused sleep apnoea treatment, disappeared, had a couple of strokes and a heart attack, and then returned to ask to try CPAP therapy after all. It's better to be late than never.

Most men will often come out in defence for many weeks or even months (or if they're embedded even longer!). But eventually their defences will come down.

What if the patient doesn't feel tired?

Amazingly, and we don't know why, some sleep apnoea patients do not feel tired during the day. I've had patients who had five sleep apnoea episodes a night and feel exhausted and other patients with 50 episodes a night but don't report sleepiness.

Like many things around sleep, the reason why this happens remains a mystery. But tiredness is also relative term. What is 'tired' or 'exhausted' to one person is not to another, just like the pain threshold varies from person to person.

It's also possible to learn to live (however uncomfortably!) in challenging conditions over time. Some people simply don't know (or cannot recall) what feeling refreshed and energized feels like after a good night's sleep, so cannot say when they feel tired.

If someone is a reluctant sleep apnoea patient anyway *and* they don't feel tired, it can be an even bigger challenge to persuade them that anything is wrong.

A patient who I'll call Tom, was such a case. Tom is a successful, high flying, busy businessman who snored. So, his wife complained and eventually, years later, he arrived at our clinic, grumbling about it being a complete waste of his time. He didn't feel tired, so how could he have sleep apnoea?

Tom was surprisingly sensible, however. He listened carefully to the evidence after his sleep study. He listened to the clinically proven risks to his health and immediately agreed he'd do something about it. He needed a CPAP machine, even if he wouldn't necessarily feel the benefits physically, he understood his body needed it.

This no doubt saved his life as it helped with an underlying lung condition that he also got treated for.

Even the loudness of snoring can be a relative term, depending on the sensitivity of the person listening.

When a younger couple arrived in our clinic together the girlfriend complained of her boyfriend's horrendously loud snoring. We did a sleep study on him, but he didn't have sleep apnoea, indeed he wasn't even snoring! So, the girlfriend got upset and assumed we hadn't done the study properly.

Eventually we did a test on the girlfriend's hearing and discovered she had hyperacusis, a condition which causes extreme sensitivity to sound. This meant even the buzzing of a fluorescent light was torture to her. It also meant her boyfriend's breathing sounded like horrendous snoring when it was nothing more than a gentle sleep sound.

Case study: Husband versus wife perspective – Steve and Katy

Steve, 60, snored so loudly his wife refused to share a bed, but he didn't want to go and see his GP. So, his wife Katy asked the GP to pay a home visit.

Katy

Steve's snoring was so loud we only shared a bed for the first five weeks of our marriage!

As soon as we had kids his snoring worsened, as there wasn't much time for exercise, so he put on weight.

Looking back over 20 years, it's hard to work out what came first for Steve, the anxiety, depression, weight gain or poor sleep.

All I knew was my husband was really struggling. He was always tired and would be crotchety with the kids.

At one point, I remember feeling so sleep deprived from having the kids too, that I thought: 'I can't stand this anymore!'. Some days it felt so hard to keep going.

Steve's snoring affected everything we did, including what holidays we could go on. We had to find accommodation with separate rooms. We also had to buy a bigger house so we could have separate rooms. Everything in our house seemed to revolve around trying to sleep through the sound of Steve's snoring.

After a few years of this, I felt desperate for Steve to see a doctor. But he refused. His reasoning was because the GP only had appointments during work hours, he did not want to take a day off work for it.

In Steve's case I think he had a negative attitude to seeking medical help because he was depressed too. Everything felt pointless and hopeless, so why bother looking for help? I believe some men don't like to seek medical help because they do not like to look weak. I have other male family members with this attitude. But in Steve's case it was his bleak outlook that affected everything, including helping himself.

Luckily, I knew our GP through a work association, so I asked him personally if he would intervene and come to see Steve for a home visit. Things were that bad. Thankfully, Steve agreed to meet him, and the GP immediately said his symptoms pointed to sleep apnoea. In the end we had to pay for private treatment as the NHS waiting list was so long.

From day one the CPAP machine made a huge difference to Steve; I saw this myself. He slept better, and the relief was huge. He could finally get the rest he so desperately needed.

Twenty years on, we still sleep in separate beds, but we don't mind. There is nothing more important than sleep for us.

Steve

After I got married, we didn't share a bed for long. I snored loudly and had restless leg syndrome, so would often wake up Katy, thrashing about.

By the time our second daughter arrived in 2000, we were both struggling, especially as our new baby cried non-stop. So, Katy started to sleep in a separate bedroom. Yet I even disturbed her behind a wall! I often woke up, shouting, because I dreamed of being smothered.

I tried gadgets such as the magnetic nose rings and nose strips, although I felt resistant to trying new things. Early on in our marriage, I did see one doctor who diagnosed a deviated septum, and I even had surgery twice including rhinoplasty and 'turbinate trimming'. Both operations were very painful to recover from and made no difference to my snoring. Everything felt hopeless.

I even considered taking part in a study that suggested singing can help tighten up the soft palate and prevent snoring.

When Katy suggested I go to a sleep clinic I didn't want to. I can't explain what lay behind my resistance, perhaps it was anxiety. So, in the end she got a doctor to pay me a visit instead.

Thankfully our local hospital had its own sleep clinic, and eventually, Katy persuaded me to get a private referral. I clearly wasn't well.

I was invited to stay overnight which to my surprise, turned out to be fun! The room involved sleeping among lots of tech and various monitors which I found really interesting.

Straight away I was diagnosed with sleep apnoea, I had 16 breath-holding episodes an hour and was prescribed a CPAP machine.

This was before they were accredited by NICE which meant the machines were cumbersome and large, but I knew I had to try.

For me, the CPAP machine wasn't a 'cure all'. I also find nasal strips help. I also had to take magnesium and look at other things to help me, like making sure my room was well ventilated. I also came across a device called a Zeez, a pebble like electronic device which you placed under your pillow. It emits electromagnetic signals like theta and delta waves like the brain does when you enter a deep sleep. The idea is the brain will be encouraged to mimic these waves and help you drift off into a slumber. Whether it's a placebo or not, I don't know.

I believe sleep can be quite complicated to 'get right' for some people and I accept this is me. But the rewards are everything, it affects everything, your mood, your outlook and of course your relationship.

Chapter six

A woman's world

'On one of our first nights together I woke up apologizing for my snoring and he pulled out two earplugs he had worn to bed so he could hear what I was saying.'

Amy Poehler[33]

When we opened our clinic only 20% of our patients were women but this figure has doubled to 40% because the word has spread that we help people sleep, be it man or woman!

In my clinical experience, women make the easier patients, who are far more open to seeking medical advice. Almost all female patients attend their sleep clinic referral willingly, listen to the diagnosis with interest and are compliant with the therapy. Even if they are initially embarrassed about snoring, they quickly understand the need to put their health first.

However, the difficulty for many women is getting their sleep apnoea symptoms taken seriously in the first place and get the referral.

Gender bias

Women find it harder to get their sleep apnoea diagnosed, partly because it's seen as a male problem and many ladies do not fit the common 'criteria' most GPs look out for. This often includes having a wide neck and of course being male or middle-aged.

Plus, many women struggle to gain access to NHS healthcare or have their symptoms taken seriously regardless of what their condition is. In one UK government study of 100,000 women, a shocking 84% said there had been times when they were not listened to by healthcare professionals.[34]

Most modern medicine is designed for the 'average man' (as much of life is!).[35] For example, women who have had a heart attack have far lower survival rates simply because their symptoms present differently to men and so they are often missed. (FYI, female heart attack patients exhibit fewer common symptoms, e.g., not chest pain but indigestion, shortness of breath and back pain).

Sleep apnoea can also present differently in women.[36] Women are less likely to report snoring (although almost all do) and more likely to complain of daytime tiredness, lack of energy, insomnia, mood swings and morning headaches.

In my experience, a woman can't often rely on her male partner to notice signs of sleep apnoea either e.g., snoring or episodes of breath holding. This is because men are not as observant or are deeper sleepers themselves.

Also, women often put everyone in the family but themselves first. I have met many female patients who were so focused on persuading their snoring male partners to seek help, they didn't stop to think of their own health. And so, their own sleep apnoea gets missed.

Plus, sleep problems in women are more common anyway and can ebb and flow over their lifetime. This can be due to hormones, child rearing (for example, breastfeeding and getting up during the night for babies and children). Society has coined the term 'baby brain' for women who become forgetful after giving birth. But this overlooks the fact that a woman is often suffering from constantly interrupted sleep by a baby who is crying or needs feeding. Perhaps we should acknowledge 'baby brain' is a likely result of acute sleep deprivation. Also, women are more likely to experience anxiety so lying awake worrying can be part of this.

Sometimes I have diagnosed the male partner first and then the female partner has realized she might struggle with sleep apnoea too and decided to get a sleep test herself. I have many couples with 'his and hers' CPAP machines who compare the number of apnoeas they had in the night, every morning. It can get quite competitive at times!

Sleep fact: The peak age for women to suffer from sleep apnoea is 65 years old, ten years later than men.

The snore shame

'I don't snore, I purr.'

Anonymous

While men tend to brush off their snoring or turn it into a joke, women tend to feel embarrassed they snore at all. Loud snoring is seen as unfeminine and something to ignore or avoid talking about.

This was the experience of one of my colleagues, Shamina. Despite spending all day treating patients for sleep apnoea, she had no idea she had sleep apnoea herself! It was a family holiday that changed everything. Shamina explained:

'We went away as a family to stay in a hotel and the kids were all arguing about who would end up sleeping in the room with me. That was when the penny dropped my snoring might be a problem. My son already complained at home, telling me I snored loudly through the wall.

My husband used to call it my "roaring" and pop into the spare room when it grew too loud.

I never said anything as I couldn't help it so would laugh it off. I was embarrassed too. It's human nature to ignore things if they embarrass you. Even though I worked in the clinic, dealing with sleep apnoea all day, I didn't spot myself as a potential patient.

Instead, I put my snoring down to other factors, for example, I often snored after a bit too much wine so assumed it was that. However, when the kids bickered badly over who faced losing a night's sleep because of the noise I made, I felt terrible and wondered if I should get it investigated.'

Shamina's issues began after she put on weight following the need for painkilling medication for a back issue. She became constantly exhausted, and it was only after I suggested doing a sleep test did she find out she was having 28 episodes of apnoea an hour.

That put her in the severe OSA category that needs treatment. Shamina quickly got kitted out with a CPAP machine and this helped her regain her energy and life.

I often find female patients only discover they snore after going away with friends such as on a hen do. It's very often other people, women usually, that gently point out the noise. A loud apnoea snore is often deep throated and rather masculine sounding, not something ladies want to shout about. The snorer's reaction is often to be mortified.

But snoring is a great alarm system to wake up a female patient to a big health problem that's easily fixed.

The pregnant snore

Sleep apnoea and snoring is very common among pregnant women, especially in the third trimester after weight gain. All pregnant women should be screened for sleep apnoea in my view, because it could save both mothers and babies lives.

Pre-eclampsia is a high blood pressure condition women are more likely to develop in the second half of the pregnancy, and also involves protein in the urine. It can cause complications in pregnancy and is a danger to both mother and baby, sometimes fatal. This affects around 0.5% of all pregnant women.

Over the last few decades, studies have shown women with sleep apnoea are at higher risk of chronic hypertension, which raises the risk for pre-eclampsia and this in turn raises the risk of premature births.[37] There is also a link between sleep apnoea, hypertension and diabetes in pregnant women.[38] Yet I do not get any referrals of pregnant women.

There is so much we simply do not know when it comes to sleep apnoea and pregnancy because, once again, so little research has been done. It would be my advice for any pregnant women who has a family history of sleep apnoea or who has other symptoms (such as loud snoring and excessive tiredness) to get herself tested as soon as possible.

We should be offering fast track NHS sleep apnoea tests for these women because by the time they wait for a routine NHS sleep study the baby will have arrived. However, when I've suggested this my colleagues in gynaecology it's often greeted with a blank look.

For this book we asked The Royal College of Obstetricians and Gynaecologists for a comment on their stance on the subject of sleep apnoea and pregnant women. This was their reply: 'Unfortunately we are at reduced capacity and therefore will not be able to support facilitating your request. Apologies for any inconvenience.'

Menopause or sleep apnoea?

Unfortunately, insomnia is very common in menopausal women due to the decline of hormones oestrogen and progesterone so around 50% suffer from sleeplessness at some point. It's thought around only 0.6% of pre-menopausal women suffer from sleep apnoea. But this figure shoots up post menopause to 47% to 67% of women, according to one major sleep study in the US.

More women in the US are obese which is why these figures are so high, but such is the obesity crisis growing in the UK, we're only five to ten years behind and so we can expect figures to rise here too.

Frustratingly for female patients, many symptoms of sleep apnoea cross over with perimenopausal symptoms. They include tiredness, exhaustion, brain fog, trouble sleeping, anxiety, depression, weight gain, etc., which makes diagnosing the conditions separately even harder.

So where do menopausal symptoms begin and the sleep apnoea symptoms end? A woman can only find out after a sleep test!

Exhausted, depressed and struggling to get help, is a common scenario for many menopausal women so it's little wonder many leave the work force in droves around this time. In a recent parliamentary report,[39] BUPA found that 900,000 women in the UK left their jobs due to menopausal symptoms. That's a scandalous waste of talent and ability.

Many will have faced discrimination at work and have been met with little sympathy or help for their symptoms. How many of these women also have sleep apnoea? We simply don't know because sleep apnoea is so under diagnosed but my guess is it is a huge proportion.

That's thousands of women leaving the workforce when their careers could have probably been saved with sleep apnoea treatment. Many of these ladies will have 20 or 30 years' work experience behind them and be a huge loss to their industry or company. That's a big toll society is paying for being essentially misogynistic.

The same Parliamentary report also quotes Dr Nighat Arif, a GP and specialist in women's health and family planning, who devastatingly describes a 'misogyny within medicine when it comes to women's health', which led to the 'normalization' of women's pain and menopause symptoms. She spoke of the need for institutional and social change in relation to the value placed on women's health.[40]

Sad sleep fact: Stars Wars actor Carrie Fisher who died suddenly of cardiac arrest aged 60 had 'sleep apnoea and other undetermined factors' on her autopsy report.

Where there's sleep there's hope

Many women I have met have spent years, even decades in some cases, being diagnosed and treated for other conditions, when their primary condition was sleep apnoea.

Maxine was a colleague, who spent 25 years suffering from depression… or so she thought. She tried CBT, counselling and antidepressants but nothing shifted the low moods. I suggested she had sleep apnoea tests when she had to sign off work for ten weeks with depression, but she laughed. She'd been told for years she was depressed and couldn't imagine it could be anything else!

I gently persisted. 'Go home, put the test on and have a snooze on the sofa,' I suggested. So, she did.

The next day we discovered Maxine was having 29 apnoeas an hour. No wonder she was exhausted and low. The CPAP machine transformed her life within a few days.

She says:

'I simply had no idea it would turn things around so fast. I took up swimming again and got back to cycling. Eventually I lost seven stone in weight. I also became a nicer person, not as quick tempered, simply because I wasn't unhappy anymore. It's unbelievable that the diagnosis of depression was so wrong, for such a long period of time.'

Many women have endured tests for other conditions such as early onset Alzheimer's disease and even leukaemia before their sleep is looked at properly.

For example, Kath Hope, founder of sleep apnoea charity, Hope2Sleep (www.hope2sleep.co.uk), spent most of her adult life struggling with anxiety and depression. Her GP didn't know about sleep apnoea, and it took a chance meeting with an ENT specialist before a sleep test was suggested.

Kath has a slight build and doesn't fit the tick box of a 'usual' sleep apnoea patient e.g., being overweight or male or having a wide neck. However, Kath's mother snored and died of a heart attack suddenly, so Kath feared the worst.

Kath's experience was so profound she decided to use her experience positively and set up a charity to help other people and raise awareness of sleep apnoea. To date they have helped over 25,000 people from all over the UK.

Case study: Kath's story

When she was 49 my mum died of a heart attack. It was a terrible shock. We were very close, and every day my little girl, only a year old at the time, used to toddle across to her house, waving at her in the window. Then one day she wasn't there. Mum always snored but we had no idea back then what the cause might be.

Meanwhile, I was struggling with anxiety and panic attacks, something I had to cope with for most of my adult life. I was a busy music teacher with about 80 students so put it down to the stress of the job and being a parent.

But every 18 months or so I would collapse with exhaustion, barely able to lift my head up. I had to have loads of tests, for every illness you can imagine from leukaemia to hyperthyroidism and every single test came back negative.

By then my daughter was 16, she was interested in becoming a nurse and came across the medical term sleep apnoea. She knew I snored and had even observed my breathing had stopped on occasion when I was asleep, so suggested I had this. But I dismissed this idea, thinking it was just something outlandish she had read on the internet. Snoring didn't bother me, as I was asleep!

I had issues with my ears as well and by chance went to see an ENT specialist who suggested I was checked for sleep apnoea. My own GP had never suggested this and when I looked it up, I didn't have the typical profile, of being male and overweight.

When I turned up the at the sleep clinic, they took one look at me, being small and a low BMI and they agreed it was very unlikely. But they did the test anyway and were stunned to see I had severe obstructive sleep apnoea. All my symptoms made sense then and of course what happened to mum hit home.

I couldn't let history repeat itself, so I immediately agreed to whatever treatment plan they had, which was a CPAP machine. This wasn't easy. None of the masks fitted me however because they were designed for men's faces with thicker necks and all of them leaked air.

I couldn't give up though.

That's when I looked online for CPAP masks and spotted there were many more makes and models from America. I ordered some and found one that fitted perfectly. Overnight all my symptoms stopped, and I felt like a new person. I had more energy, felt calmer and the anxiety just lifted.

I told the clinic about the masks from America and word spread with other patients, so I began passing them on. Then I opened a shop on eBay, not to make a profit, but to sell to other people to help them too. More and more people began asking me for them, even knocking on my door during music lessons to ask for a mask. Before long I found myself supporting around 5,000 patients, single-handedly. So, I gave up the music teaching and looked into starting a charity.

Realizing there is such a need not only for these products but also for awareness around sleep apnoea,

I set up Hope2Sleep and it became a registered charity with a team. To date we support around 25,000 people.

I am so grateful, for my diagnosis. When mum was alive, CPAP machines didn't exist, so it was never going to save her. But I had the chance of treatment, so history is not repeating itself.

At the charity we get emails from people saying: 'You saved my life' or 'you saved my marriage' every single week. Sleep is such a necessity, whoever you are.

Helping people with sleep apnoea find the mask to help them achieve that deep sleep is so rewarding. I've gone from someone who had no idea what sleep apnoea was to becoming a passionate educator about the condition.

Case study: Michelle's story

Michelle, 48, went to see her GP around ten times and was refused a sleep test for many years. Only a chance conversation with a consultant in preparation for surgery led her to finally being referred to a sleep clinic.

My main symptoms were exhaustion and chest pain. I'd wake up at night feeling like someone had dropped a brick on me. Once I woke up in such pain, I thought it was a heart attack. I'd wake up with such a jolt it was like someone had punched me.

I also started snoring really loudly and as my husband was already on a CPAP machine, I knew about sleep apnoea, and he suggested I had it. But when I suggested this to the GP he didn't agree. I kept going back and forth but kept being told it was the menopause or the symptoms were connected to my arthritis or my fibromyalgia. But I knew this chest pain was different to my other pain. It just grew worse and worse. But nobody would listen.

Then I needed elective surgery and after speaking to the doctor he looked at me and said I need a sleep study. He asked for a GP referral but incredibly the GP still refused! Eventually it took five months before he agreed to do it, after the consultant himself asked him again.

Finally, I had the study done. It found I had 52 episodes of apnoea in an hour, so it was severe. It was no wonder I was tired and in pain. I felt so let down it had taken so long to get diagnosed, but once I had, I was hugely relieved. I wasn't going mad.

It took me several weeks to get used to the CPAP machine as I kept pulling my mask off in my sleep. But I persevered because I knew I had to for my health. Now I wouldn't be without it. I sleep deeply every night. I wake sometimes in a little pain from other ailments but nothing like previously. It shouldn't have taken so long for doctors to take my concerns seriously.

The numbers of women coming to our clinic is ever rising and with the obesity crisis growing in an ageing population, I expect to see more women in my clinic in future years.

My advice is for any woman, shape, or size, if you snore or feel permanently exhausted, don't delay doing the questionnaires. Then get a sleep study done if need be.

Chapter seven

Junior snorers

'It's easier to build strong children than repair broken men.'

Frederick Douglass[41]

Sleep apnoea is a condition which is relatively unknown among adults, but among children, even less so. Around 12% of children snore and at least 3% of children in the paediatric population suffer from sleep apnoea.[42] Almost all of them will end up not being diagnosed or become misdiagnosed with something else, such as ADHD.

I get only around 100 paediatric referrals per year and that's in Lincolnshire, a catchment of a 700,000 population with a child population of around 128,000.

That means approximately 1,300 to 3,800 children in Lincolnshire will have sleep apnoea and haven't been diagnosed. Scale that up nationwide and with 12 million children in the UK, that's a staggering 360,000 children who live and suffer with undiagnosed sleep apnoea.

These children will likely struggle to do well in life. They may be overweight (due to being hungrier due to tiredness) or labelled with ADHD or other behavioural issues or learning difficulties.

Tragically, children with sleep apnoea are literally sleepwalking through their educational years and their dreams of a bright future will be blighted. They will not be able to focus on lessons at school and will fall behind. Many will be diagnosed with ADHD or behavioural issues and even get prescribed drugs like Ritalin. Other children face being labelled as fat and lazy by society, when the reality is, sleep apnoea could lie behind it all.

My suggestion if a child presents symptoms such as snoring and unsettled sleep, is to simply look inside their mouth at their tonsils.

> 'I actually stop breathing, I think it's 80 times a night, because I have sleep apnoea. I've had it since I was a kid.'
>
> Shaun Ryder[43]

The tonsil test

Don't be like Shaun Ryder. Sleep apnoea can be cured and change a child's life and their life chances. Tonsils and adenoids blocking the airway is a huge factor in diagnosing sleep apnoea in children and any parent who suspects sleep apnoea should ask to get them examined.

The peak age for tonsil growth is between two and eight years old. Most children presenting with sleep apnoea show symptoms around three years old when the tonsils become enlarged and start blocking the airways, but this can happen earlier.

A big issue here, again, is educating GPs and health visitors to spot sleep apnoea in children as soon as possible. It's easily missed. Most parents do not know what to look out for either.

Sleep fact: By school age, children should not need a daytime nap… unless they are sleep deprived.

How can a parent spot sleep apnoea in their child?

Every parent knows what it's like to nurse a sick child or watch them sleep badly at night. But imagine seeing your child thrashing around in bed, struggling to breathe? It can be absolutely terrifying.

By the time I meet the mums and dads in my clinic, they will often have spent years trying to get help only to be met with blank faces from GPs or misdiagnoses.

Many will have had to provide video evidence of their child's struggle for breath. This is because during the daytime breathing issues might not be evident at all.

Sleep apnoea in children causes loud snoring very often. But they can also seem restless in their sleep, struggling, tossing and turning, sometimes gasping. It can be extremely distressing for a parent to watch. Once you have heard the sound a child with sleep apnoea makes, it's hard to forget.

Other signs at night-time could include:

- choking or coughing;
- dry retching;
- sweating at night;
- mouth breathing;
- sleep terrors;

- nightmares;
- crying;
- bed wetting.

Apnoea causes a stress event on the body, due to excessive adrenaline production caused by lack of oxygen. This can be a frightening experience for adults, let alone children. That's why children with sleep apnoea will have nightmares and often wake up crying or struggle to settle. Parents report it being almost impossible at times to calm their child back into bed.

Observing the child's behaviour during the day can be very telling too. For example, a child who hasn't slept properly will not be able to concentrate in the classroom. It would be almost impossible to sit still. They could have very poor memory and not even be able to recall what they learned the previous day. Tiredness in children manifests as being fidgety, overwhelmed by noise or light or other people, and inability to focus.

We need to experience restorative sleep in order to learn and recall our memories effectively. The REM part of the sleep cycle consolidates what we are taught during the day. You need to sleep properly beforehand to be prepared to focus for the lesson and the night after the lesson, to embed and consolidate memories.

Children with sleep apnoea do not stand a chance with learning properly if they cannot experience enough REM slumber. As long ago as 1889, the British Medical Journal reported children with poor memory and concentration issues, labelling them as 'stupid' but were they stupid or did they actually have sleep apnoea?

Whipping them out

In most cases when a child has sleep apnoea, they need their tonsils or adenoids (or both) removed. This is always my recommendation.

However, the availability of this treatment is a postcode lottery. In my county of Lincolnshire, as in lots of areas, the recommendation is that recurrent tonsilitis (seven in a year, or attacks three years in a row and documented by GP) must have taken place before a child can be referred for a tonsillectomy. If sleep apnoea is suspected, they must also have a sleep study and be proven to have sleep apnoea before this referral for a tonsillectomy. This is of course because it's dangerous to have a general anaesthetic if you have undiagnosed sleep apnoea.

But this advice does depend on how local health commissions work. Some health authorities will pay for tonsillectomies happily and others will not. Some patients will easily get access through their GP and a quick referral for a sleep test and then consultant while other parents get no support.

At one stage taking out tonsils was one of the most common operations in the country. For decades, especially in the 1960s and 1970s, doctors whipped tonsils out at the drop of a hat but that all stopped back in the 1990s.

After studies were conducted to examine how necessary this operation was (looking at statistics such as how many patients would eventually get better anyway), the decision was made to reduce the operations availability.

I agree surgeons were previously too keen to whip out tonsils at the first sign of any issue. As with all surgeries there are risks attached so no surgery should ever be done unless it's really needed. But equally GPs are now often overly risk adverse when it comes to referring patients to consultants for surgery.

The main risk factor for tonsillectomy occurs post operatively. One in 20 children will have a problem after the operation and this is usually because one tonsil starts bleeding excessively, due to infection. Why is it usually one tonsil only? Nobody knows. But this is the general case.

When this happens, it's key for the child to seek urgent help. This risk can be mitigated by educating the parents of the child to know what to watch out for after their child's operation. Any sign of bleeding in a child means they need to be rushed straight back to hospital, with an on-call ENT department specialist on standby for proper care. This is vital information to know. Parents should look up the best hospital in case it isn't the same hospital they had the initial operation in. There needs to be both an emergency team and ENT specialist available for any emergency follow-up treatment.

Sleep fact: Tonsils are larger in childhood, to help fight infection, but shrink from age six upwards.

Other sleep apnoea risk factors in children

There is evidence to suggest that 'glue ear' could also be linked with sleep apnoea. When adenoids are inflamed, this can lead to glue ear, where the middle part of the ear fills up with a sticky, gluey fluid. This problem can be persistent and require grommets, which are ventilation tubes to aid hearing.

The ears, nose and throat are all linked, as we know, so some parents with children who have glue ear should watch out for mouth breathing and other signs of sleep apnoea.

Also, children with Down syndrome have a much higher chance of developing sleep apnoea due to their shape of face and jaw. One estimate is that 53% to 76% of children with Down syndrome have sleep apnoea but only a tiny number ever get diagnosed and helped.[44] Sadly, many children with Down syndrome grow up to develop early onset dementia. There is a link between dementia and sleep apnoea and so the lack of sleep apnoea therapy could be contributing to high numbers.

Also, children with cerebral palsy and sickle cell disease are at higher risk of sleep apnoea.

A genetic link cannot be ruled out too, so if parents have sleep apnoea, it's wise to watch for signs in the child.

How do you get a diagnosis for your child?

All of the parents who come to my sleep clinic have had trouble getting a referral, so here's my advice: Go to your GP well prepared to fight your child's corner.

GPs generally have around 8 minutes per appointment so make it easy for them to understand what is happening and why you suspect sleep apnoea in your child. This means it's key to prepare evidence before you go.

First of all, record a video of your child struggling when they sleep. Take off the child's pyjama top and video the snoring and any struggling for breath. The accessory muscles, diaphragm and chest muscles may all be struggling so get this clearly on film if possible.

Keep a short sleep diary, with notes of your observations. Make note of any mouth breathing, poor behaviour, and other daytime symptoms too. Do they appear to struggle to listen? Do they often come down with lingering coughs and colds and appear congested? Do they speak clearly, or does it sound garbled? If you can, attend the appointment with a partner for extra emotional support but also to back up what you're saying.

Explain to the doctor you would like further investigation for sleep apnoea and if necessary, make the link with enlarged tonsils. Specifically, ask for the Choose and Book/e-referral system and a quick referral if a referral is accepted.

Frustration in the NHS system

Regardless of whether you're seeking a diagnosis for a child or an adult, we have to understand the NHS system is at breaking point in many parts of the country. This means it's difficult to get a GP appointment, even on the telephone at times. It can be hard to get a referral for anything, anywhere. Factor this in. It's better to be prepared for the frustration so you don't give up at the first hurdle.

Brace yourself for the frustration, delays, long waiting times on the telephone or in the surgery. Brace yourself during the appointment and come armed with information. Sadly, it is a fact of life for many people seeking medical help in the UK which is deemed 'non-urgent' but we need to keep going and be persistent for our long-term health. Preventative medicine should be taken more seriously but with such stretched services, it very often isn't.

Stick to your guns and keep fighting for a referral if you believe you need one.

Putting off getting medical treatment causes so many more problems in the long term for so many issues, not just sleep apnoea. So, grit your teeth and keep going. Get the initial appointment and be very clear about what your concerns are whether the appointment is for the adult or the child.

Sleep studies and children

Like adults, children need a sleep test to work out what the problem is. Many parents wonder how on earth medics will manage to do a sleep test on their restless, wriggly child. And it can be challenge! We do not offer tests to children under the age of five years or any children with special needs or multiple conditions because of the specialist equipment needed. Those patients would be referred to their nearest children's teaching hospital.

The tests we offer are always two-night studies. This is to allow for the children to get used to the device. We also offer good guidance on how to make it work successfully. We have had children turn off the sleep test in their bedroom because like other electronic devices they get switched off at night! But between parents and sleep specialist nurses we can get the data needed.

Case study: Charlie's story

Charlie, 44, spent years taking her daughter, Tilly, back and forth to see her GP for help with sleep issues but it took a chance observation from a health visitor to change everything.

Right from when she was a baby Tilly never slept well. She struggled to settle and couldn't drop off unless I was holding her upright. As a new mum I assumed it was reflux or that it was just normal for little babies to struggle to settle.

But by the time she was a toddler the sleep didn't improve. She was constantly waking up, then of course was exhausted during the day. She also always seemed to be dribbling or had a runny nose. We tried to limit dairy in her diet and that seemed to help a little bit, but I started to worry something was wrong. She was always mouth breathing and picked up a lot of colds and sore throats which left her really poorly.

When Tilly tried to speak, she sounded garbled, as if she was being strangled. But every time I saw my GP, to ask if this was normal, I was reassured she was still young and things would change.

Every day felt like a battle as Tilly was so tired but also her behaviour was tricky. She would get easily overwhelmed in places like soft play or parties. Then I noticed her snoring was getting worse. It got louder and louder until we could even hear it in the downstairs living room.

By the time Tilly started nursery, we began to get calls from the staff, suggesting she was being a bit rough with other children. I was upset, but also wondered if her lack of sleep made her ability to emotionally regulate harder.

I went back and forth to the GP again, but each time I was made to feel like an overly fussy new mum.

By the time Tilly started pre-school she was struggling in lessons with her behaviour and couldn't cope with the busy atmosphere in the lunch hall at lunchtime.

Finally, an eagle-eyed health visitor picked something up. She noticed Tilly sitting very close to the TV when she came to visit.

'Does she always sit that close?' she asked. I confirmed she did.

'Has she had a hearing test?' she queried.

Tilly had the test as a baby but not since. We arranged for one and it showed she had glue ear. This explained so much. She wasn't being badly behaved, she simply couldn't hear what was going on most of the time and background noise was torturous for her. Then we got an ENT referral.

The consultant looked into her throat and announced: 'There is the answer to all the problems!'

Her tonsils were graded 4, which meant they were very big and blocking her throat. On giving her health history and my observations, he concluded Tilly had sleep apnoea. He booked her in for an adenotonsillectomy operation to remove her tonsils and adenoids and put in grommets.

A month before the operation, Tilly became unwell again with a bad throat, so I took her back to the GP for a check-up. This time the doctor looked inside her mouth and let out a scream when she saw Tilly's tonsils. 'She needs to go straight to A&E!' she said.

Thankfully after getting antibiotics, Tilly recovered and just before her fifth birthday, she had her operation.

It was like a miracle afterwards. Doctors told us it would take at least a week to recover, but within days Tilly was cheerfully playing in the garden, chattering away. What's more, she slept for 12 hours that first night afterwards and has done every night since.

Tilly is like a different child. So much happier and calmer. It's so sad that sleep apnoea isn't diagnosed for most children. A simple operation can change a life and I wonder how many children out there won't get the help they need.

Part three

A mad, tired world

Chapter eight

Waking up to a sleepless society

'Time is a created thing. To say: "I don't have time" is to say, "I don't want to".'

Lao Tzu[45]

Tackling any sleep disorder can be a challenge but the truth is our cultural attitude towards sleep doesn't make it any easier. As a society we simply don't take sleep seriously enough.

Sleep deprivation is a global health crisis with around 40% of adults and children in the UK suffering from sleep issues. It doesn't matter what age, class or gender, sleep loss affects us all.

Our society measures our value regarding our productivity, mainly economic productivity. We are told to get through the working day no matter what.

'Get an alarm clock and get up early!'

'Be on time for work or school!'

Being busy is what is valued in our society, not being well rested. While we are bombarded with public health messages such as:

'Get your five portions of fruit and veg a day!'

'Drink eight glasses of water!'

'Don't smoke!'

'Cut down alcohol units!'

'Exercise more!'

We rarely hear about the importance of having 7–8 hours of sleep a night. When was the last time you saw a billboard or TV advert explaining why sleep matters? Taking time for deep restorative sleep has never been a public health message, despite there being so much evidence that it should be.

Artificial tinkering with our body clocks

Every single year the clocks go forward with the 'daylight saving' hour kicking in at the end of March. But studies prove there is a marked increase in the number of heart attacks, strokes and even a 6% increase in fatal car accidents. This is due to our body clock being suddenly shifted by only 1 hour!

If we also factor in the technology we use every day, then it should come as no surprise our bodies and minds are changing, and not for the better.

The stark rise is obesity particularly in the young is now a global problem and seems to correspond with the uptake of this new digital world. One study notes: 'The prevalence of mobile phone overuse is high in areas of social exclusion and is associated with sleep disorders, school failure and obesity.'[46]

Is this any surprise if we are spending at least 6.5 hours using our phones and other devices? This is a sedentary activity.

Many of us blindly accept tiredness as a fact of life. There are so many reasons for exhaustion including excessive work hours, family commitments, stress, illness, the 24/7 culture with constant access to emails and social media via our phones. And of course, undiagnosed sleep apnoea or other sleep disorders such as insomnia.

People often talk about being exhausted, being busy, trying to catch up on sleep at the weekend, or a longing for a holiday. In many cases being sleep deprived is viewed as a badge of honour, something inevitable if you lead a successful life.

Many of us don't even recognize we are sleep deprived. We simply stagger through the days, exhausted, never considering how things could and should be different. Certainly, we don't talk about the impact this has on our long-term health.

How often do we reach for a coffee or tea, to help power through the afternoon? Needing caffeine is a clear sign of sleep deprivation, but it's shrugged off.

The many reasons why sleep isn't valued certainly includes an economic one. Sleep cannot be sold for a profit. There's no money to be made if you're well. We are apparently a clever species yet are the only beings who force themselves to stay awake when tired to the detriment of our own health.

Our family cat, Dusty, is a professional sleeper. All he does is eat, chase mice, and sleep for hours and hours. My daughter derives a lot of comfort from watching him curled up, soundly asleep. The cat has encouraged my daughter to become an Olympic sleeper, just like I am. In our house we all try and get our 8 hours in every night, no matter what. My son even did a school project on gaming and the impact gaming at night has on sleep deprivation and being able to do cognitive tasks. As much as he loves video games, he quickly understood how it impacted the effectiveness of his study the following day at school.

I've taught my children that sleep matters and getting the amount needed provides rewards for both the body and mind.

My wish is that every family in the UK appreciates sleep as much as we do. Our nation would be much healthier and happier for it.

Tick-tock time bomb

As a sleep apnoea specialist, I also foresee the health time bomb we face as a country if we continue not to take sleep and sleep apnoea seriously.

This is for several reasons. The first is that the UK population is a rapidly ageing one. Let's unpick the statistics. People aged 85 years and over was estimated to be 1.7 million in 2020 (that's 2.5% of the UK population) and this is projected to almost double to 3.1 million by 2045 (that's 4.3% of the UK population).[47]

The second reason is that obesity is rising, which means diabetes will rise and so will cases of sleep apnoea. By 2040, there will be 21 million adults who are obese, so therefore sleep apnoea cases will rise too.

The toxic mix of being an overweight, sleep deprived, ageing population means cases of dementia and diabetes will explode. Just think of the knock-on effects of the chronic illness in store for those people.

Sleep fact: Already around 40–50% of those with dementia experience sleep apnoea symptoms which accelerates their condition, a third of those with high blood pressure have undiagnosed sleep apnoea already too. And those are the conditions we know about![48]

There is already four million people in the UK with sleep apnoea, so this is set to skyrocket in the next decade. Sleep apnoea, dementia and diabetes are all closely linked and all cost huge amounts to treat on the NHS and social services is already massive. As a society offering free healthcare, we simply cannot afford to ignore sleep apnoea any longer.

This lack of vision when it comes to sleep, and medicine is clear madness.

If sleep is the best medicine, why is it not a branch of medicine?

Actually, these are starting to form across the country with different specialists involved, from Chest Physicians, ENT Surgeons, Anesthetists and Neurologists.

Every part of the human physiology fits into a medical specialism. We have carved up medicine for each chunk of the body; cardiology for hearts, pulmonology for lungs, renal for kidneys, ENT for ear, nose, and throat, etc., but sleep straddles them all. Sleep doesn't fit neatly into any category of body because it affects all categories.

When it comes to sleep apnoea, even more confusingly, the symptoms cross over with symptoms from many illnesses and conditions. Tiredness and brain fog can be signs of menopause or depression, for example. What's worse is that many people with diabetes, who are obese, hypertensive, have cardiovascular problems, etc., might have developed sleep apnoea first before their illness but it was never spotted.

As one of my nurses said, when she spots obese people on mobility scooters in the high street who are likely to have a range of health issues, she wonders how many have been screened for sleep apnoea? Probably very few.

Raising awareness and education is key for putting sleep at the forefront of our health agenda. But to do this our societal attitude towards sleeping needs challenging at the same time.

Case study: My campaign to raise sleep apnoea awareness

My goal is to raise awareness of sleep apnoea and one way this is being is done is with an all-party parliamentary group. Our aim is to spread the word about sleep apnoea and the devastating impacts it has on people's health and lives.

Dementia is one related time bomb we have discussed because it's such a big-ticket item. All political parties can see the dementia tsunami heading our way, but what are they going to do about it? I am hoping to persuade those in power to take sleep apnoea seriously, increase public awareness with proper campaigns and make apnoea therapy more easily available on the NHS.

While we don't have a cure for dementia, we do have a 'cure' for sleep apnoea.

I think the Lords are the appropriate people to speak about sleep apnoea because after all, it's a place that's famous for people nodding off!

In all seriousness, the House of Lords is a place packed with the brightest brains from around the country, if we can't save these ones what hope is there for the rest of us? These are 700 people from all walks of life, many who have achieved extraordinary things over the course of their long lives.

Many Lords are devoted public servants with decades of experience who want to continue serving their country for as long as possible. This means they'll want to keep hold of their brain cells in their twilight years and sleeping well is one way to help this happen.

A couple of the Lords have spoken privately about having sleep apnoea too. One of them was recently diagnosed and got a CPAP machine. 'I've seen the light!' he told me, as if it was almost a religious experience.

Another Lord confided that he often nods off during the day and experienced brain fog but he'd yet to join up the dots. Of course, sleep apnoea is a likely cause.

That's why I have suggested *all* Lords in the house get screened for sleep apnoea. A bold request but it could transform their lives for the better. And if they see how easy the therapy is to use, perhaps they'll legislate for more people on the NHS to get the same care.

If sleep apnoea screening saves the country's brightest minds, then it can save the rest of us.

The macho sleep culture

In our mad, tired world, sleep is viewed as something to minimize and indeed, if you're able to get by on little sleep, something to boast about. This starts from the top of society down.

Think of these common sayings:

'You snooze, you lose!'

'Wake up sleepy head!'

'I'll sleep when I am dead!'

That last quote was an album title from musician Warren Zevron, who died aged 56 from cancer (although of course we don't know if this was related to lack of sleep).

This powerful message that sleeping is for the weak often comes from our leaders. Over the last century many political figures have boasted about not sleeping. The idea being, they are so mentally strong and tough, they can cope without sleep – a necessary biological function.

We don't boast about not needing to eat or use the loo, so why sleep? Once again, it's down to the myth that not sleeping creates more time for productivity and this is linked to our 'success' in life.

Tony Blair talked about needing melatonin pills when his body clock was out of whack, while a former number 10 aid even spoke out about Gordon Brown's lack of sleep and how it could affect judgments.

Jonathan Powell said: 'I would always rather work and vote for a leader who sleeps well than one who wants to be woken up all the time.'[49] I agree. The idea that anyone can run a country on a few hours' sleep should seem ridiculous and not looked upon as a strength.

It's not just those at the top of the political game that don't value sleep. It's businesspeople too. Jack Dorsey who invented Twitter (now X) boasted how he only got a few hours' sleep because he was so busy; Richard Branson says he can get by with only a few hours in the sack; and Apple CEO Tim Cook says he gets up at 3.45am to check emails. This makes me feel exhausted just thinking about.

There's some glamour involved in believing you can get by without sleep too, with artists and pop stars bragging about their ability to avoid it. Keith Richards once claimed he stayed awake for nine days in a row. Whereas movie star Tom Cruise boasted: 'I go without sleep,' as he publicized his latest film. But lack of sleep will only make life feel *Mission Less Possible* (sorry!).

We are conditioned to believe to get to the top of your profession, forgoing a good night's sleep is inevitable. Indeed, if we're not prepared to feel tired, we might not even be working 'hard' enough.

The madness is that the complete opposite is true. We need deep restorative sleep for our brains to function fully and perform at our physical and mental peak. It's why serious athletes include sleep in their training schedules before a competition.

Studies show if we're tired our work productivity dips by around 30% and we struggle to focus with memory problems and poor emotional regulation.

This is almost without exception. People who claim to only need 5–6-hours sleep (or anything below the 7–8 hours), are doing themselves damage. Science proves this.

Of course, there may be a tiny number of exceptions to this rule. Humanity's great bell curve teaches us there will always be exceptions. For example, the world record for breath holding while free driving is an extraordinary 24 minutes, but this is very exceptional and does not mean almost anyone else can do it.

It's the same with sleep. The next time someone tells you 'I only need 5–6-hours sleep' they'll be functioning below par and facing long-term health consequences.

Machoism in medicine

Even those working in the medical profession don't always take sleep seriously. When I became a surgeon in the early 1990s, and we all worked on a rota system where we worked on call every other night. Often, we clocked up around 100 working hours a week. After a 72-hour shift, I barely knew my own name due to exhaustion! This naturally played havoc with circadian rhythms but none of us ever complained about feeling fatigued. We didn't dare. It would be seen as a sign of weakness and incompetency.

In a male-dominated industry such as surgery, the macho sleep culture still rules. Sadly, this applies even for medics who have more awareness around the science and importance of sleep.

But sayings like, 'Sleep when you're dead' are unbelievably stupid, because if you *don't* sleep properly, you will die sooner and probably in a more unpleasant way.

Caffeinated culture

'Coffee is a language in itself.'

Jackie Chan[50]

Caffeine is one of the most widely used psychoactive drugs in the world. It's estimated a staggering 80% of the world's population consumes some form of caffeine daily. Yet few people understand it's seismic effects on our lives and on our sleep.

A molecule in caffeine blocks adenosine, a chemical found in human cells that gradually builds up during the day to reach a height in the evening that causes sleepiness. However, caffeine blocks adenosine temporarily, so that's why after the initial buzz of after a tea or coffee we often experience a slump, because the excess of adenosine floods back in. That's payback time for the artificial boost of energy.

Caffeine affects our body quickly, reaching a peak within as little as half an hour yet it stays in our bodies for many more hours. Just 500mg of caffeine (that's about four cups of fresh coffee), can feel the same as a low dose of amphetamine but the more you drink, the more you need as tolerance builds up.

Caffeine boosts our mood, makes us temporarily more alert, increases concentration levels but the flip side is the withdrawal. This makes us irritable, lethargic, headachy and less sharp. At worse, too much caffeine can make us feel shaky, anxious, nauseous and unwell. Yet most people view coffee and tea as completely harmless.

Indeed, tea is part of our UK national identity with approximately 100 million cups of tea being drunk every single day.[51] We offer to 'put the kettle on' in times of emergency, in times of stress or to welcome people into our homes. Who doesn't love a cuppa! But how much of this caffeine is interfering in our sleep?

The recommended 'safe level' is 400mg per day, that's about four cups and limiting use to stop sleep interference is recommended.

While many of us can enjoy a lovely cuppa first thing, and I am among those, it's important to understand how long caffeine remains in the system. It's 12 hours. So, if you drink after midday, you face having a powerful stimulant in your body in the early hours of the morning. Caffeine interferes with the REM sleep cycle, so if you drink it in the late afternoon chances are you won't sleep well.

Coffee shop take-over

Caffeine is a substance in the world that's hard to avoid. Walk down any high street and you likely don't have to go far to stumble across a coffee shop. Starbucks started with one shop in Seattle over 40 years ago and now has a staggering 32,000 branches in 78 different countries. Whatever happened to making a quick cup of instant coffee at home? Today, coffee is part of a shopping culture.

Costa coffee is the UK's largest coffee chain, with over 2,600 UK stores. CEO, Jeffrey Young, of the Allegra Group who runs the chain, describes coffee shops as being a 'crucial part of the UK's social fabric'.

At around £3.35 a cup, it could be said coffee does more harm to our wallets than our health. Recent research also reveals that drinking moderate amounts of coffee may be more likely to be beneficial to our health than harmful too.[52]

But it's what lies behind the coffee shop culture that's more worrying. Coffee is a stimulant, and its normalization could definitely reflect how tired we are as a nation. If coffee is needed habitually to get through the day, it's a major sign of not getting enough kip.

Is it a coincidence that our sleep deprived 24/7 culture has exploded at the same time as coffee shops? I think not.

Cuppa facts: Two billion cups of coffee are drunk world-wide every day, that makes it the most popular drink in the world.[53]

Energy drinks

'I was drinking so much coffee and Red Bull, it screwed me.'

Frankie Boyle[54]

Soft drink sales have gone down, but studies have shown that sales of energy drinks which are packed with caffeine have shot up by 155% between 2006 and 2014.[55]

Worryingly, many of these energy drinks are targeted to young people with bright colourful packaging and funky adverts. Even social media influencers are pushing their products. For example, popular YouTubers and influencers promote Prime energy drink which has high quantities of caffeine, the equivalent of two espressos.

These drinks promise to improve concentration or give a much-needed boost (or 'wings' according to the Red Bull adverts, a drink that has a 25% market share).

But there's growing evidence these drinks are bad for young minds and bodies. High in sugar and caffeine, studies have linked these drinks to obesity and even heart arrythmias.[56] In some cases, deaths have been linked with young people guzzling these drinks that give them a temporary buzz but little else.

Time for a nap?

Instead of having a caffeinated drink, would a short nap be better? Studies reveal how a short daytime nap can help improve our cognitive skills (and make life feel less exhausting).[57] But that's not how the world works for most of us.

A teacher, James, told me how coffee brewing equipment in his staff room was seen as a 'must have' because 'everyone knows it's caffeine that powers teachers through the day'.

'I go home with a lot of work to catch up on, and often don't finish until 9pm, leaving little time to wind down before bed. Instead of questioning how many extra hours of overtime we do (for free usually!) it's normal for everyone to feel tired by the afternoon. Virtually every single member of staff drinks numerous cups of coffee and tea, especially in the afternoon. It's totally normal. When people need caffeine to function, maybe we should question why?'

I agree. What if we made sleep and rest time the priority rather than another cuppa?

This is happening in some parts of the tech business world, where 'nap pods' have been installed in offices to encourage 40 winks. Nike and Google are among the big employers who appear serious about wanting to encourage rest time.

Proctor and Gamble even changed their lightening system to dim lights in the evening to aid production of melatonin.[58] But big business still has a long way to go before sleep deprivation awareness is anything like mainstream.

There are far more vending machines selling caffeinated drinks in offices than nap areas!

Wake up to blue light

There are 3.8 billion smart phones in the world, and research published by Virgin Mobile discovered phone users receive 427% more messages and notifications than they did a decade ago.[59]

Wow. That's a lot of extra information for our brains to process every single day. It's little wonder that phone use affects our moods. Scrolling on social media is also known to increase the production of dopamine, a feel-good chemical released after sex, great food, exercise or a social interaction. Even spotting the little red dot indicating a phone message gives a hit of dopamine. That's an addictive experience for our brains.[60] So, we alternate between getting hits of dopamine and feeling angry, low or shocked by 'doom scrolling' all the bad breaking news. And we do this for hours and hours. According to 2023 research from Data Reportal, the average screen time for users around the world aged 16 to 64 – across different platforms and devices – is 6 hours and 37 minutes.[61]

Imagine if we swapped our hours scrolling and staring at our phones for sleep or winding down for decent sleep?

Few of us can be without our phones and I admit my own is like an extension of my arm. I don't even like being without a backup charger either – just in case. In fact, I have two chargers on me when I leave the house!

But with our dependence on the smart phone, we need to also understand what the blue light they emit is doing to our bodies and how this affects sleep.

What is blue light?

Blue light is everywhere! It comes directly from the sun and even fluorescent light bulbs. In fact, one third of all light is blue light. It can have health benefits too, for example, it can be used for helping clear acne from the skin or for those suffering with seasonal affective disorder (SAD) because the light boosts our mood.

However, with all the technology in our homes, we are exposed to more blue light than ever before because all of our digital devices are backlit with blue light. This includes laptops, tablets, smart phones, Kindles and LED TVs. Often with these devices we spend hours on them per day, often at close range.

Our eyes have a cornea and a lens which can filter out some harmful lights, including UV, however we cannot filter out blue light. In fact, even our skin absorbs this light, and this interferes with our ability to make melatonin, which is the hormone that makes us feel sleepy.

In the natural world, we would be woken by the blue light of the sun, then feel sleepy when the red and orange hues of sunset descend because melatonin is triggered by these colours. However, if we are staring at blue light into the evening, our bodies do not make enough melatonin, so our sleep cycle gets disrupted.

It takes our bodies 90 minutes to overcome the blue light exposure. So ideally, we need to lay down the devices for at least an hour and half before bed. Yet, how many of us are this disciplined? Although the jury is out over how much damage blue light does to our eyes research proves it interferes with our sleep.

The market for blue light filtering products is growing. There are screen covers and glasses for sale, but this is the equivalent of putting a filter on a cigarette. The best thing to do is not to use your device at all at least 2 hours before bedtime.

One mother came to me at the clinic with her 14-year-old daughter who suffered from terrible insomnia. Doctors had examined her, she'd had brain scans, body scans, kept a sleep diary and nobody could work out what was wrong. She simply couldn't drop off to sleep quickly or easily.

Her tiredness was affecting her ability to concentrate at school, so her grades suffered. Her mood swings were awful. It was hell for her and for her poor parents. But within a few minutes of our consultation, it was clear what this teenager's issue was. Blue light!

This young teen didn't go to bed until near midnight, and often used her smart phone right up until then. If she couldn't sleep, she went online, scrolling away to while away the hours. The amount of blue light absorbed wreaked havoc with her sleep cycle. By putting strict boundaries around her use of the gadgets, this young girl's sleep cycle quickly improved.

This is all relatively new tech that is affecting the younger generations in particular because they are growing up with this stuff. It's like techno crack for children.

The harm these devices can cause is evidenced by litigation in the US already with the makers of Fortnite paying out $520 million for violating federal law by exposing children to a myriad of online dangers.[62] The long list includes harassment, bullying, psychological trauma, sexual predation and invasion of privacy. All these factors of course, will interfere with sleep.[63]

I sound the alarm now as we do not know what health consequences, as a species, we are all about to suffer with as a result of this new way of living our lives through tech. Make no mistake that these companies intend to use all their resources to get you and your children hooked on the dopamine hits we get off these interactions no matter the price. Currently the companies involved seem happy to pay the fine and move on without any accountability.

I cannot understand the inaction of UK and other European Courts as compared to US but perhaps we will catch up with the legal and harmful consequences of this tech later on. I'd like to see any settlements go towards research and development into sleep science studies. Something good should come out of all this.

Tech and its effect on us are a big issue and our children are guinea pigs. Once we start messing around with dopamine levels who knows where it leads to.

When I was a child, the TV went off at 10pm, and that was it. If I wanted to stay up it was a case of using a torch under the duvet. Now my son has a laptop, a smart phone, video games and the TV. If I want him to go to bed by 11pm, he must switch it all off by 9.30pm and be made aware of the effect these gadgets and blue light has on his body and mind. None of this is easy for parents to navigate, never mind the children.

Sleep fact: Modern 'time' was not invented until 1884. This was when delegates from 25 countries met in Washington and signed a resolution stating that the meridian passing through Greenwich was the zero meridian. They subsequently established a global system of timekeeping to define modern time, which we still use today.

Our natural body clock

'Early to bed, early to rise, helps makes a man healthy, wealthy and wise.' That's an old proverb but doesn't work if you're a night owl or indeed a teenager. It was also made famous by Benjamin Franklin, a clergyman and one of the founding fathers of America who probably wanted to encourage economic productivity in the new world.

Science backs up the popular belief that some of us are naturally early risers (morning larks) while others can happily stay up late into the night (night owls).

But studies also reveal if you are a morning lark, you're at a significant advantage compared to the night owl because of society's insistence on an early morning culture. For example, both work and school start early in the morning.

I notice this difference at home. I am a morning lark and feel fresh and ready by 7am to start work whereas my wife, a night owl, cannot hold a conversation before 10am but livens up around 10pm – when I am winding down and ready for bed!

Research of the brain, led by the University of Birmingham found that participants whose 'natural' internal body clock prefers late nights and late mornings have lower resting brain connectivity in many brain regions which is linked to the maintenance of consciousness.[64] This lower brain connectivity is associated with poorer attention, slower reactions and increased sleepiness throughout the hours of a typical working day.

So, that means half of the population who are night owls struggle with early morning starts for work or school. Once again this makes no sense for productivity or learning if half of us can't function properly for at least part of the day.

It's also not a myth that teenagers need more sleep than adults. This is a scientific fact and not some excuse because they're lazy or love lounging around in bed.

A teenage brain is still in development and there's evidence to suggest it doesn't become fully developed until the mid or late 20s. Research has also revealed melatonin levels drop in the mornings but stay high at night in teen bodies especially. This is why younger people can stay up clubbing, etc., and often struggle to wake in the mornings.[65] I see this in my 13-year-old son, whom I also cannot converse with most mornings!

These adolescent sleep patterns are at direct odds with how schools, colleges and universities expect young people to function. Most class lessons begin at 9am or even earlier, meaning a groggy start for many children.

In an ideal world our daily lives should work around our body clocks, not the other way around. This might sound unrealistic but it's something we're waking up to.

Society trying to change for the better

In 2022, a state law in California took effect to prevent the start of college classes before 8.30am and no earlier than 8am for middle school children, to allow for the difference in the teenage circadian rhythms and their need for more sleep.[66]

If young people are tired, they're not ready to learn, but later on in the morning their minds will be more receptive, so this makes perfect sense. There was another surprising result of this.

Researchers analysed car accident statistics involving adolescents in Fairfax County, Virginia, for two school years before and after the introduction of later school start times. Incredible results show that the crash rate in 16–18-year-old licensed drivers decreased significantly from 31.63 to 29.59 accidents per 1,000 drivers after the delayed start time.[67] Tweaking the hours to match our natural body clocks can make the world a safer place as well as making it easier to learn. Sadly, there are no plans to change school or college hours in the UK.

Chapter nine

The huge cost of little sleep

'The reason laziness is rarely pushed as a lifestyle option is down to one simple reason: money. There are fortunes to be made from active lifestyles. Gyms charge fees. But no one is going to make money out of sleep. It is free.'

Tom Hodgkinson[68]

What does the government care most about? Money! That's why in my ongoing campaign to raise awareness of sleep apnoea, I highlight the economic cost to our society that sleep deprivation causes.

Sadly, car crashes are one way of adding up the cost. A staggering one in 25 of us will fall asleep at the wheel, without even knowing it. This is because our bodies enforce sleep upon us if we are sleep deprived.

Driving can be a monotonous activity and can involve staring at the same strip of road for miles, often in a heated vehicle, and often around the same speed. So, it's easy to 'switch' off because it's quite hypnotic. Drifting off to sleep may last just a few seconds, but when you're travelling at speed that's more than long enough to cause a serious crash.

One study found that people who have had less than 4 hours sleep and get behind the wheel are as likely to be involved in a car crash as a drunk driver. The motorists studied shows that the mistakes they were making, putting them at risk of a car crash was the *same* as if they were 1.5 times over the legal alcohol limit.[69]

Because most of us don't know if we have sleep apnoea, this means there's potentially hundreds of thousands of people driving around at risk of having a 'microsleep' without knowing it. We can choose not to get behind a wheel if we have had a drink, but if we have a sleep condition we don't know about, then there's no choice.

One of my patients, Mohammed, was one such driver. He lived with undiagnosed sleep apnoea for years. Here he describes what it's like to fall asleep behind a wheel.

'One minute I was driving along an A road, then I completely zoned out, lost track of all time and experienced a strange "falling" sensation, like you do in a dream. Then suddenly I came to again. It was very scary because I was behind a wheel of a vehicle and on a dual carriageway. It only happened for a matter of seconds but instantly I knew it was long enough to veer off the side of the road. The incident shook me up and made me wonder what was happening to my body.'

This is scary stuff. It led Mohammed to give up using his motorcycle and only drive when he had to. At the time he was unaware he had sleep apnoea, and it took several more years before he got a diagnosis.

Sleep fact: Some driving companies have included dashcam cameras to monitor their employees for signs of exhaustion and an alarm is then emitted to wake them up.

How sleep apnoea therapy can save lives (and money!)

Where I live and work, in Lincolnshire, most people need a car to get around. The area is rural, and the public transport service is rubbish. Unless you fancy waiting at a bus stop for several hours then you'll need a car to get from A to B.

Other environmental factors make the county a perfect storm for road accidents due to sleep apnoea. First, the county has rural roads which means they are badly lit at night, and often have deep watery ditches running alongside them. This means people often sadly drown if they crash. Another unique factor is the high proportion of obese people who live in Lincolnshire. Around 66% of the total population are obese – the highest number in Europe and as we know, obese people are more likely to have sleep apnoea.

This toxic mix of poor roads, reliance on cars and high prevalence of sleep apnoea means car accidents are tragically common.

In 2000, the Lincolnshire Road Safety Partnership was set up to try and reduce the costs of these accidents. Of course, the human cost is impossible to quantify, but the economic costs are also shocking. A fatal car accident, for example, costs over £1.8m.

This is factoring in the services of police, ambulance, coroner, enquiries, road closures, and of course the economic losses from the poor person who got killed too. A serious crash costs £200k and even a slight accident is over £15k. That's a huge cost to our economy, let alone someone's life.

It is known that those with obstructive sleep apnoea has a 7–12 times increased risk of having a road traffic accident. It's notable here that this risk drops by a phenomenal 83% if a CPAP machine is used as therapy.

Therefore, having a sleep service in an area like Lincoln where sleep apnoea is diagnosed and treated saves huge amounts of money and lives. Is there proof of this? Yes, there is.

Our sleep clinic in Lincoln first opened in 2005, and that year there were 69 fatal car crashes in the area. Over the following seven years these crash figures went gradually down as more people came for help and more sleep apnoea therapy was prescribed.

By January 2012, we had over 2,000 residents on CPAP and only 39 fatal crashes, saving about £54 million a year. The number of fatalities had therefore almost halved since our Sleep Disorders Centre opened. How amazing considering that there were no major road developments or other factors that could have caused such a dramatic reduction.

Are these figures due to the use of CPAP machines and other therapies? Yes. The police and local community agree. After every crash, investigators can work out whether driver tiredness was a factor by eliminating all other factors. For example, they examine the road condition, no evidence of braking or evasive manoeuvres, condition of the car and any signs of drink or drugs in the driver. If no other evidence points to the reason for a crash, then tiredness can be a reasonable assumption.

CPAP facts: There was a study which showed a near 50% reduction in healthcare costs from using CPAP too. Two hundred and eighty patients with OSA were compared to a control group over a five-year period. Before the use of CPAP, the cost to the health service was around £2,720 per year and this was reduced to £1384 per year.

Lost productivity

It's not only money and lives that are lost to lack of sleep. Hours and hours of work productivity is at stake if employees are tired. This should also wake up companies and the government to the importance of sleep!

Ground-breaking research carried out by a family nurse practitioner in Florida, Dr Clelia Lima, revealed that a big company could save an estimated $136m in lost productivity if they screened high-risk employees for severe sleep apnoea. The study examined the top-level managers at this huge (unnamed) company and many of these employees were middle aged and obese and therefore high risk of OSA. But of course, around 80–90% of sleep apnoea remains undiagnosed.

The same research revealed that work productivity dropped by a whopping 30% if someone has sleep apnoea. If this study, known as the Lima study, was reflected across all global companies, then it's clear what a mammoth loss of wealth sleep apnoea causes.[70]

Sleep fact: Did you know, if you declare you have sleep apnoea when you set up a pension annuity, you can claim around £12,000 more.

In 2017, the Centre for Disease Control and Prevention in the US declared that 'insufficient' sleep is officially a public health problem after a study examining the economic burden of insufficient sleep across five different OECD countries, including the UK.[71]

The report states that *insufficient sleep can result in large economic costs in terms of lost GDP and lower labour productivity.* It also highlights the proportion of people having less than the recommended amount of sleep is rising due to the 24/7 culture.

One recent UK survey of 1,000 people found that almost half of employees admitted they often turned up to work feeling too tired to work. Three in ten people admitted to having had an accident, making serious mistakes or feeling very stressed due to tiredness. Worryingly these included high-risk employees, and also includes those working in the construction industry and manufacturing.[72]

The dangers of a sleepy work force

I'd wager that all of us have slept badly at some point, gone into work, struggled to focus, and muddled through the day. Luckily for many jobs tiredness doesn't cause harm, but in jobs which involves the responsibility for others, it can be deadly. Tiredness is a major contributory factor in some of the UK's and world's biggest disasters. Here's a list of just a few of them:

Zeebrugge ferry disaster: In 1987, 193 people lost their lives when a ferry capsized near Zeebrugge. In the subsequent court case, it was heard how one of the staff fell asleep and didn't hear the signal to close the bow doors of the boat, which flooded with water and caused the ship to sink.

Chernobyl: In 1986, the nuclear reactor power plant in Russia exploded, causing (over the next few decades) around 4,000 deaths. Investigators concluded that 13-hour shifts led to fatigue and human error that contributed to the tragic accident.

The Challenger shuttle: In 1986, the NASA space shuttle exploded within seconds of take-off tragically killing all seven onboard. Human error due to exhaustion was to blame with some employees admitting to the inquiry they'd had only 2 hours sleep the night before take-off.

Clapham rail crash: In 1988, 35 people tragically lost their lives when a packed commuter train crashed into the back of a stationary train. Among the technical failures, the enquiry afterwards also blamed a long hour's culture where excessive hours were not limited for rail staff.

We can never know how many of these employees might have had sleep apnoea. What we do know however is that screening for the condition could save lives in the future.

Shift work

One reason for excessive tiredness in the workplace is shift work, which plays havoc on our circadian rhythms. Around 12% of the UK work force are employed in shift work in many fields including NHS staff, manufacturing, transportation, security, entertainment and service industries.

Between 10–30% of shift workers report sleep disorders, with either trouble nodding off or waking up too early.[73] This is because our bodies love routine for sleep and with shift patterns, the routine changes every few weeks.

Not only is it bad for our cardiovascular system, but long hours may also increase the risk of depression and anxiety. Night shift work is linked to an increase in the risk of breast, prostate, and colorectal cancer, as well as dementia.[74]

Many highly skilled fast-paced jobs in medicine involve shift work. A&E staff must work 12-hour shifts during the day and then swap to night-time shifts in three-week periods. Incredibly, half of junior doctors also admitted they've had an accident or near miss travelling home from a long shift.[75] Every year a few junior doctors even lose their lives to accidents due to fatigue. What an absolute tragedy.

Other countries, such as Norway, recognize the health risk due to shift work and even factor in extra pay to compensate. But what is being done in the UK to combat this fatigue at work? In many jobs there are restrictions in place to limit the number of hours a shift worker is allowed to work. For example, in the NHS, the minimum rest period for a worker is 11 hours within a 24-hour period. But for many other jobs, in the gig economy for example, there are fewer rules in place.

When it comes to shifts it would be safer and better for our bodies if patterns did not change so frequently and if employers had a better understanding of this. There should be greater legislation in place to protect employees from the effects of sleep deprivation not only to improve productivity but to save lives.

Sleep fact: In 2013, a bank employee in Germany dozed off at his keyboard and accidentally turned a minor transfer into a 222-million-euro order. The exhausted banker meant to transfer just 62.40 euros from a bank account but instead 'fell asleep for an instant, while pushing onto the number 2 key on the keyboard' – accidentally making it a 222,222,222.22-euro mistake. The bank discovered and corrected the error shortly afterwards.[76]

A dream to save lorry drivers

Discovering how screening for sleep apnoea reduces the risk of road accidents led me to look at the haulage driving community.

Lincolnshire is known as 'the nation's breadbasket' because of The Fens and surrounding areas includes much agricultural land, providing a fifth of the nation's crops. This means there are around 25,000 haulage lorry drivers working in Lincolnshire, many driving through the county to deliver goods nationwide.

In my estimation, one in six HGV drivers could have sleep apnoea, and of course in most cases it will be undiagnosed. How did I reach this figure? Well, many lorry drivers hit the high-risk criteria, being male and overweight (often due to poor diet on the road). That's a lot of sleepy drivers in charge of ten-tonne vehicles hurtling along our narrow country roads.

Armed with this knowledge, I decided to approach haulage companies to see if they would consider screening all their drivers for sleep apnoea. Many were interested to hear what I had to say. We got as far as talks with major lorry companies but talks fell apart. But I understand the company's predicaments around taking responsibility for their driver's potential sleep apnoea.

It's legally tricky for the big corporates because any results which are found cannot subsequently be denied. It means that if drivers find out they had sleep apnoea but doesn't comply with proper therapy and then had a crash the company could be held liable for corporate manslaughter.

In theory, screening lorry drivers is a simple solution to a large problem and many lorry drivers themselves were open to the suggestion of being screened too, so I hope one day sleep apnoea screening will become standard practice. You could apply the same logic to tube drivers, train drivers and coach drivers. The more damage you could do depends on the size of the vehicle and how many passengers you are carrying.

The potential cost to people's lives and our society is far too great.

Case study: Adrian's story

Adrian is an RAF engineer who specialized in fixing military aeroplanes, but he struggled with sleep apnoea for years, without knowing he had it.

His wife complained of his snoring, and he tried every anti snoring device out there, but nothing worked. He always woke up feeling exhausted, often suffering from headaches, and then feared making mistakes in his job.

I've always snored. Ever since I was two, after an accident where I broke my nose, but I simply got used to it.

Once we were staying in a hotel and overheard the residents staying three doors down say: 'Did you hear that awful snoring last night?' It was me!

Of course, the snoring also affected my relationship with my wife Michelle. She would often have to get up and sleep in the spare room. But she snored sometimes too, so we were quite understanding to each other about the situation!

I used to get the odd migraine but gradually they grew worse and worse. I started struggling to focus at work, which was not ideal, as my job is to fix electrical equipment on aeroplanes.

Luckily everything is rigorously tested because occasionally I would make the odd mistake, and not understand why. This began to affect my self-esteem as I wondered what was wrong with me. I also used to need a nap at lunchtime when the exhaustion took over.

Then my elderly dad was diagnosed with sleep apnoea and got a CPAP machine. Mum suggested I also got checked out. Both Dad and I snored loudly, so it was bit of a family joke.

In the end it wasn't the snoring that made me make a GP appointment it was the headaches that forced me to take time off work.

Luckily, I very quickly got a referral to the sleep clinic. Even in the waiting room I realized I had a problem when I fell asleep and woke myself up three times by snoring. After the test, moderate sleep apnoea was diagnosed, with 26 apnoea episodes happening every night.

After the diagnosis, I got the CPAP machine and everything instantly improved. I never need to nap and my sharp focus at work has returned.

My work can still deploy me anywhere, maybe not anywhere with a tent, but anywhere with an electrical plug for my CPAP machine! I cannot believe I struggled for so long.

The sleep deficit builds up

It's easy to understand we need the golden 7–8 hours sleep and hope for the best, but the reality is small seemingly incremental lifestyle factors adds up minutes of lost sleep. For example, commuting, smoking and eating sugar can all cause loss of sleep.

Some of these factors are surprising. The CDC study from America (Why Sleep Matters, the Economic Costs of

Insufficient Sleep) reveals the full list of lifestyle factors that stop us from sleeping:[77]

- **Obesity:** Those with a high BMI on average between about 2.5 minutes to 7 minutes less per day than those with a normal BMI.
- **Smoking:** Current smokers sleep on average 5 minutes less per day than non-smokers.
- **Sugary drinks:** People consuming more than two sugary drinks per day sleep on average 3.4 minutes less per day than those with less consumption of sugary drinks.
- **Physical activity:** People performing less than 120 minutes of physical activity per week sleep on average about 2.6 minutes less per day than those reporting to do more than the recommended 150 minutes of physical activity per week.
- **Mental health:** People with medium to high risk of mental-health problems sleep on average 17.2 minutes less per day than those with low risk of mental-health issues.
- **Commuting:** People commuting between 30–60 minutes to work (one way) sleep on average 9.2 minutes less per day compared to those with a 0–15 minutes (one way) commute. Heavy commuters travelling more than 60 minutes to work (one way) sleep on average 16.5 minutes less per day than those with only short commutes.
- **Financial concerns:** People with financial concerns sleep on average about 10 minutes less per day than those without concerns.

Other factors include being an unpaid carer, having unrealistic time pressures, working irregular hours, having children and marital status all cause us to lose sleep. Our gender matters too as men sleep on average 9 minutes less than women.

A few minutes here and there of lost sleep seems negligible but adding it up is a real eye opener.

The study gives this example: *To put this into perspective, an employee who works irregular hours, commutes 30–60 minutes to work (one way) and is exposed to a set of different measures of workplace psychosocial risks, such as unrealistic time pressures, sleeps on average about 28.5 minutes per day less than an employee that has regular working hours, commutes only up to 15 minutes (one way) and is not exposed to psychosocial risk factors at the workplace. This equates to over 173 hours of lost sleep per year.*

The study goes on to point out that mortality risk shoots up by 13% if you sleep for less than 6 hours a night compared to someone who sleeps for 7–8 hours. Even someone sleeping 6–7 hours a night has a 7% higher mortality risk (and this is for all factors including fatal car accidents to cancer to heart disease). This makes sobering reading.

Frustratingly, our NHS healthcare system makes treating sickness the priority rather than preventative medicine. For example, diabetes costs 10% of the entire NHS budget and with spiralling rates of obesity this will only rise. How is this sustainable? It isn't.

But how much money is spent on *why* people become obese? From educating people on how to cook without using ultra processed foods to raising awareness of how lack of sleep is linked to feeling hungrier, there is so much need for more awareness. There are so many ways we could educate people on making better choices for their health. Sleep is inevitably part of many solutions for many diseases. With the dementia and obesity/diabetes/sleep apnoea tsunami set to overwhelm us, we shouldn't kick these issues repeatedly into the long grass.

The cost isn't just economic, it's a cost to our lives and our loved one's lives.

Part four

Sleep, the best medicine

Chapter ten

How to win the snore wars!

'Sleep is the eternal fountain of youth that you can dive into daily.'

Dr Michael Oko

Getting a good night's sleep is the key to health, happiness and longevity. It really is that simple. But achieving this can feel difficult, if you or your partner snores or if sleep apnoea is suspected. Getting a test booked for sleep apnoea can feel challenging especially for a reluctant snoring partner. But it needn't be this way.

Very quickly sleep apnoea can be tested for and effectively treated. It can be cured for many people. In this chapter we explain everything you need to know for making the pathway to help easier.

Persistent snoring should be treated as the ultimate alarm system for potential sleep apnoea. Not everyone who snores will have sleep apnoea (roughly one in five snorers have it), but it needs investigation via a sleep study test as soon as possible. So how do you book one?

There are numerous sleep clinics in big cities like London, but far fewer in other parts of the country. When I opened our Snore Disorders Centre in Lincolnshire, it was the only clinic in the area. Anyone who had suspected sleep apnoea had to drive a 4-hour round trip to clinics in other counties, which was dangerous madness.

Finding a sleep clinic without a long waiting list is a postcode lottery. Some clinics have waiting lists as long as 18 months. That's a long time for your body to become damaged by OSA. But knowing how the system works is one effective way to navigate the minefield for your own benefit. The Sleep Apnoea trust website offers a link to every single sleep clinic in the UK.

Summary of steps to getting help:

- Fill in the Stop Bang and Epworth questionnaires.
- Make an appointment with your GP and take the completed questionnaires with you.
- Take your partner along if you have one (both of you will benefit if this gets sorted).
- Ask specifically for the 'Choose and Book' system also known as e-referral for a sleep clinic appointment.
- Find a sleep clinic with the shortest waiting list/ or nearest one to you.

If there are not any appointments available within 40 weeks, you can try the Patient Initiated Digital Mutual Aid System (PIDMAS – find via your local Integrated Care Board for contact details). You should be contacted by your local hospital, and you should be able to request to be seen in a clinic with a shorter waiting list. Also asks if the potential clinic offer virtual services. These are far quicker and more convenient than in-clinic appointments which involve travel.

Theoretically you could have a referral from a GP and a sleep clinic appointment within weeks, but as previously stated, be prepared to factor in frustrations of the current NHS system.

If you are diagnosed with moderate or severe sleep apnoea, you will be offered the gold standard for treatment, the CPAP machine, which is fully funded on the NHS. If this therapy doesn't suit, then other treatments are available and explored in Chapter eleven.

The goal is to reduce the sleep apnoea episodes to as close to zero as possible, or at least to under five per hour.

However, the wait list for the initial sleep study can take months and you need a GP referral to get a sleep clinic appointment in the first place. Communicating with a GP effectively can also be a battle. Read on for the best strategy for picking your battles to win the war.

Step-by-step from GP onwards

Before you go and see your GP arm yourself with the relevant information. A GP has just 8 minutes allocated time per patient. Make their job easier by being very clear in your own communication to get the result you want.

It is down to the discretion of the GP to make the referral to the sleep clinic, so they need to be convinced this is the correct course of action. Some GPs won't have sleep apnoea on their radar. This is because GP training varies, some younger doctors will have had it, other older GPs might not have. Therefore, be ready for every eventuality.

Many of my patients told me it took them years to get a referral because they went to their GP 'for snoring' and faced blank looks. 'My wife sent me here,' is what many male patients end up telling their baffled GP, before they're shown the way out. Many men are simply not articulate when it comes to being advocates for their own health issues.

For others it doesn't come naturally to complain or bang on about health issues. Many people put up with tiredness for years thinking it normal or minimize their poor health symptoms out of habit.

For others their sleep apnoea symptoms are mistaken for other causes, which are tested for and if nothing is found, then they don't pursue it. Some patients get diagnosed with say, high blood pressure, and are prescribed lifelong medication.

Others feel anxious about asking for tests in the first place, 'in case of what they find'. Ignorance might seem bliss but not when it comes to sleep. By now we understand sleep apnoea will catch up with everyone who suffers from it.

So, the time to bite the bullet and get a sleep study done is always *now*. If you're vague and woolly about what your symptoms are when you go and see your GP, you're unlikely to get a referral.

The first step is to fill in the questionnaires both Stop Bang and Epworth Sleep scale in Chapter three. Once these questions are answered, print them out and book your GP appointment. Also, if you have a partner, take them along too. Your partner can back up your evidence and provide emotional support. This is the person who shares your bed (or sofa, or car, if you have the propensity to fall asleep during those activities too!) and can share their observations during the appointment.

If the GP *still* says no to a referral for a sleep test or does not agree with your suspicions of sleep apnoea, then ask for a second opinion with another GP. This is a right every NHS patient has.

If your GP agrees to refer your case to a sleep consultant, then the next key request is to ask specifically for the 'Choose and Book' system or e-referral system.

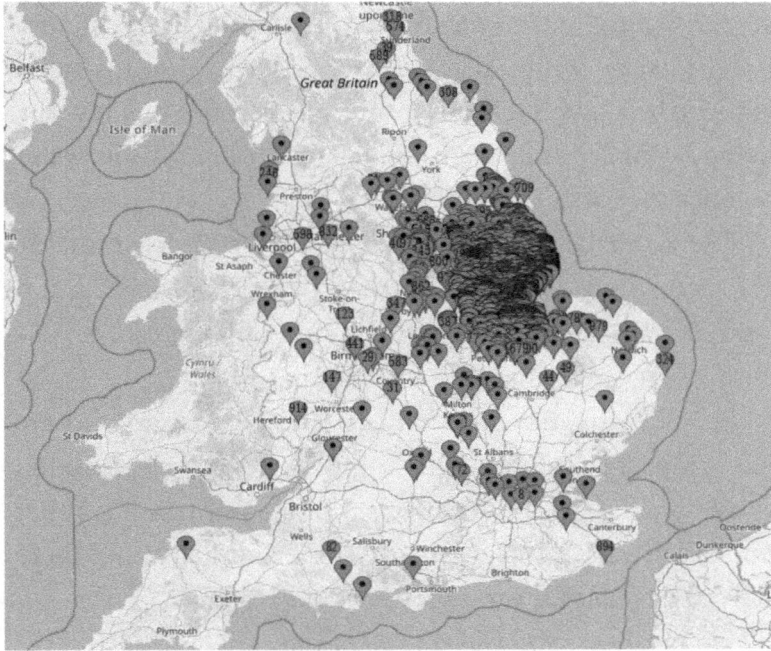

Figure 10.1 The patients treated by Dr Oko's clinic spread all over the UK

This is an online NHS system which allows you to choose a hospital or sleep clinic and book an appointment at a date and time that is convenient for you.

Via this system you can research waiting times, find out how far away the clinic is and if they offer online appointments. The wait times will vary. The wait for my clinic is currently six weeks but others could be several months or longer. It's possible to choose a clinic that does online appointments miles away if it suits if the waiting list is shorter.

What if I don't want to wait for NHS treatment?

Get the ball rolling anyway if you can afford it. Every month trying to sleep with untreated severe sleep apnoea is not a risk worth taking. Not only could it save your life, but any therapy can also transform the quality of life for the better too once the exhaustion lifts.

The scandal of long waiting lists for sleep disorders on the NHS is ongoing. In some instances, patients are waiting two years for care. In my opinion this is not offering care, that is offering a promise that's not delivering.

People with diabetes or high blood pressure who are not being checked for sleep apnoea face their condition worsening as sleep apnoea affects the outcome of both. Other statistics are stark too: a person is one and half times more likely to develop cancer if they have sleep apnoea.

We need to go to the source of the problem. Fixing the apnoea can transform a patient's life but it's not happening for enough people fast enough, or in many cases at all. So, if you can pay for it, go privately, and find a sleep clinic directly through self-pay system. But make sure the clinic is a run by a consultant with GMC registration.

Ideally you should look for a sleep consultant who also works for the NHS as we are regulated by the GMC which gives more assurance of dealing with an honest broker, and who is liable for monitoring. Only those doctors and specialists who are registered must demonstrate knowledge is up to date and are fit to practise. You can search doctors by name on the General Medical Council register at www. gmc-uk.org.

Insurance minefield

If you have private medical insurance, take a good look at your paperwork. The policies for many insurance companies don't make sense when it comes to sleep disorders. For example, the biggest insurance company in the UK, BUPA, won't cover sleep apnoea, yet places like BUPA Cromwell offer sleep studies. Effectively they will cover patients for conditions like strokes or heart attacks, but not sleep apnoea (which can cause both).

Other insurance policies vary. For example, our clinic has arrangements with AXA, Cigna International, Simply Health and every other insurance company except for BUPA. But their policies vary wildly, for example, AXA will cover the first consultation, sleep study and follow up but won't pay for a CPAP machine. Cigna International pays for the whole lot in the US, partly because they're an American company and they get more bang for their buck over there. Depending on where you live in the world there will be some local funding mechanism for diagnosis and therapy – whether it be self-pay, insurance, co-payment or state funded.

Big companies providing private medical insurance for all their staff is a good example of a system that's not necessarily set up in the patient's true interests. So why do companies offer it in the first place? Two reasons: 1) it's because private insurance is a tax write off; and 2) it makes the employee feel as if they are valued.

In reality, private medical insurance is a bit of your wages which is not directly financed as money in your bank account but offset. At face value it looks like the company cares about their employee's health, but really offers limited lip service.

Part of working with the all-party group is trying to bring about change and make sleep studies and sleep apnoea therapy easily available to everyone. We want to persuade the NHS to increase provision and hopefully this will also persuade insurers to accept they should cover sleep apnoea even if they argue it is preventative medicine. There is very good evidence to suggest that if insurance companies invested in CPAP for patients, there could be a saving of 50% of health costs over the following two years. So that's a saving of 100% of the money spent within four years! Clearly, the current system is a false economy. Watch this space.

Studying your sleep

So, you've navigated the GP, opted for 'Choose and Book' or 'e-referral' and now your sleep clinic appointment has arrived. What happens next?

Many sleep clinics offer remote appointments (e.g., online via Zoom). Remote medical appointments reduce the obstacles for accessing medical healthcare considerably but also still provides effective healthcare. One Australian study reveals how patient satisfaction was the same if an appointment was made remotely for CPAP prescription and aftercare, as it was if the patient was face-to-face. Currently appointments via telecommunications are efficient and save everyone time and money.[78]

During the appointment a sleep clinic consultant or nurse will take down patient's details, look at their medical history from the GP, then organize a sleep study which can often be done at home. The study is a good diagnostic tool but isn't the whole picture. I take sleep study data with a pinch of salt because the whole patient history must be evaluated, including psychological and medical alongside it. This is in case anything else is missed.

For a lot of people too, even doing the study can be a challenge, because they don't sleep well that night knowing they're being studied! This sometimes creates a false reading, well known as the first night effect. If this is suspected, then request it is done over two nights.

What happens in the sleep test?

The sleep test device consists of a chest belt that monitors breathing, an oximeter that fits on a finger to monitor heart rate and oxygen saturation and a tube with little prongs to go up the nose to monitor air flow. The device also has a body position sensor, so we know if the sleeper is on side, tummy or back. Some people only have really bad apnoea if they are on their back. So that means we can advise additional therapies, even simple ones, like sewing a tennis ball in the back of your t-shirt.

Most tests can be carried out at home. The sleeper goes to bed with the device on, gets the best night's sleep possible and mails it back. Afterwards is a follow-up consultation, where the results are discussed and what is the most likely useful treatment.

Sleep apnoea is measured by AHI (Apnoea Hypo apnoea Index). A pause of breath must occur for at least ten seconds, and we count them over the course of an hour. The depth of breath is also monitored, so a shallow breath would be around 50% of a normal breath. If the test comes back normal, it's a straightforward discharge. If the sleeper does not have apnoea but snores in a harmless way, there are suggestions on how to overcome that later in the book. But if sleep apnoea is diagnosed, the next step is to discuss what treatment will be preferred and most effective.

Treatment options for sleep apnoea

CPAP therapy is what is always prescribed for moderate and severe sleep apnoea. The aim is getting the episodes of apnoea as close to zero as possible. The other option is a mandibular device which sits in the mouth like a mouth guard or, as a last resort, surgery.

If CPAP is chosen, mask fitting and options will be discussed with a nurse. All my nurses are specialists and some of them are on CPAP themselves so they understand how daunting and psychologically challenging the idea of sleeping with a mask can be.

After fitting, the support remains in place. Many people need to make numerous mask tweaks before they can drift off easily, while others take to it like a duck to water. When appropriate, nurse specialists can visit a patient's home to help set them up. Some patients need help with sorting out where the plug socket needs to go, or how to log their machine onto the Wi-Fi etc. Many sleep clinics offer services to help the process of the initial set up run smoothly.

If a patient is still having trouble, they can also always contact a nurse for more help. Once the machine is up and running, a doctor should have remote access to make sure it's monitored and working correctly and can make machine adjustments as required remotely.

After six months a follow-up appointment will be made. This is the shelf life of an average mask and around then it is likely to start to leak air. Sometimes patients tell our nurses they don't want to waste money replacing their mask. '*I don't want to waste NHS resources*' some say if they haven't noticed a leak. But this attitude is a false economy. If the therapy is not used properly at the optimal level, then the risks from the sleep apnoea will increase. The cost to the NHS of a stroke or heart attack is much higher than the cost of a new mask!

I have devoted a whole chapter to CPAP therapy in Chapter eleven.

Sleep expert cowboys

These days, anyone can build a website and claim to be an 'association of' or 'specialist' or 'expert' in any medical condition. There are numerous companies that claim to offer sleep help or make promises to help stop snoring.

A tell-tale sign of a cowboy is to see if a medically trained person is running the website. Look closely at who the site is registered to and where they are registered. Be especially wary again of clinics that are run by consultants who are not GMC (General Medical Council) registered or companies offering machines that are not properly tested.

Be wary of sleep clinics offering treatments without any monitoring at all. Some clinics now offer home tests and then equipment, which needs to be signed off by a doctor somewhere along the chain but if a patient is not being monitored then how do they know the equipment is working? It doesn't make sense not to monitor the efficiency of your machine either.

I always advise my patients to look at their data via the App daily and then they can have an informed discussion with me. It is possible to buy a CPAP machine (e.g., the Air Sense 10) and download an app (MyAir app) to examine progress. This is a bit like being a diabetic and having the kit to monitor your blood sugar levels. It can be useful but still, I would suggest also being monitored by a medical professional too.

Realistic costs of CPAP

If you have had a private clinic study done, then you will need to pay for the therapy equipment afterwards. The clinic should be able to recommend machines to use. A sleep machine costs around £500 to £700 and needs replacing every three to five years. The mask is costs around £100, needs replacing every six months and the tube costs £30 and needs yearly replacing. Filters also need replacing when they discolour which depends on the background pollution levels in the room.

As mentioned, ideally a trained medical professional who monitors any device prescribed for regular check-ups will make sure your therapy is working as it should. Tweaks might need to be made for maximum efficiency.

If you're going to the trouble of wearing a mask at night, then having a properly trained medic to advise along the way should be the goal.

Grey areas

Like most things in life, diagnosing a sleep issue is not always clear cut. As we have explored there can be other medical reasons for sleep issues. Can there even be other reasons for struggling to breathe during sleep that's not OSA or central sleep apnoea? Yes!

Upper Airway Resistant syndrome is where there is some kind of blockage in the throat but instead of having an apnoea, the person powers through, forcing breaths. This requires an excessive amount of energy. They end up snoring like a pig and feel like hell because they're not getting enough oxygen.

This condition causes all the features of sleep apnoea but is not sleep apnoea and a sleep study could reflect this result. Therefore, they're less likely to be offered NHS treatment because the 'computer says no'.

But they shouldn't give up. CPAP or the mandibular device can still be an effective form of therapy for Upper Airway Resistance, and this can still be provided by a sympathetic clinician.

I always say the patient and their medical history and current symptoms should be believed rather than any squiggly lines on a report. The sleep test is only ever part of the story and is reflective of that particular night(s) only.

If a sleep test is done and shows it's a negative but the symptoms still present, then a patient needs closer investigation.

Case study: My sleep story

How I was diagnosed with moderate sleep apnoea.

When I started work as a surgeon 33 years ago, I acknowledged the importance of sleeping well.

The phrase 'Physician Heal Thyself' is an ancient proverb from the Bible but has real meaning because a doctor who is responsible for the lives of others should take responsibility for his own health.

Often, I had little time to wind down before bed especially after performing dramatic surgeries such as a tracheotomy (which gets the adrenaline going!). Dropping off to sleep fast was something I had to master.

However, by my 40s I had put on some extra pounds and my wife began to complain about my snoring. Usually, it occurred on my back or after I'd had some drinks. But my wife got annoyed enough for me to test myself using the sleep test.

I understand all too well the affect sleep apnoea has on the body. I had also struggled with high blood pressure for the past decade and knew sleep apnoea contributes to this.

My job is a cerebral one and, keen to hang onto my brain cells for as long as possible, I wanted to find out if I had sleep apnoea.

So, I conducted four or five tests on myself which revealed my breath-holding episodes were hitting the target for moderate sleep apnoea. I tried masks until I found one that fits and got a prescription for a CPAP machine. It really wasn't a problem. Now my breath-holding episodes have reduced to 0.5 per night or less.

As a doctor, I am naturally interested about my own health outcome. But I urge everyone else to be as curious to their own. There are so many gadgets out there to help monitor our health. Preventative medicine should be everyone's goal.

Being medically fit for driving

The DVLA is rightly concerned about people sleeping at the wheel, similarly to alcohol.

One of the biggest concerns from many patients (especially men!) before a sleep test is that a diagnosis of sleep apnoea (obstructive sleep apnoea in particular) will cause them to lose their driving license. This is especially a concern for those who drive for a living. This does not need to be the case. The official DVLA website states:

You must tell DVLA if you have:
- *Confirmed moderate or severe obstructive sleep apnoea syndrome (OSAS), with excessive sleepiness.*
- *Either narcolepsy or cataplexy, or both.*
- *Any other sleep condition that has caused excessive sleepiness for at least 3 months – including suspected or confirmed mild OSA.*

You must not drive until you're free from excessive sleepiness or until your symptoms are under control and you're strictly following any necessary treatment.

The fine for not telling the DVLA is up to £1,000.

This sounds draconian, but in practise is a very simple process to adhere to. It's also important to note that some people have an elevated AHI but are NOT sleepy, hence they do not have the syndrome only sleep apnoea. The key word here being 'excessive sleepiness' which is so hard to define for individuals. Most people will say 'no' if they're asked if they fall asleep while driving.

It's easy to follow the DVLA website links to give the details and then the sleep clinic will guide you on what you need to do with compliance.

If you have been diagnosed with moderate or severe sleep apnoea, then you must use a prescribed treatment for at least 4 hours a night (70% of the time), that's 4 hours using the CPAP machine or a mandibular device. Obviously, the WHO guidelines suggest 7–8 hours a night for sleep, but the DVLA don't want to be overly harsh, so 4 hours is accepted as the minimum needed.

In practice, a handful of people out of thousands of cases couldn't achieve 4 hours of sleep, 70% of the time. The 4 hours doesn't even have to be consecutive. You can do 2 hours and 2 hours, or 3 hours and 1 hour in a 24-hour period and the machine will log 4 hours for you, and you only have to do it Monday to Friday.

The better your CPAP machine is monitored by a healthcare professional the better outcomes you get. As a sleep doctor I can get remote access to a patient's machine and therefore tell if someone has used it. So, for example, if one of my patients had a driving accident but their data proves he was using his CPAP machine then he can say to authorities that fatigue wasn't the cause.

Case study: Linda's story

I thought a sleep apnoea diagnosis would definitely stop me from flying... it didn't!

Linda's husband Mike would stay awake, nudging her when she stopped breathing in her sleep for years, but both assumed her tiredness was down to being a busy mum who also cared for a disabled son. Until a sleep test proved otherwise.

I'd struggled with exhaustion for years and Mike often watched me struggle for breath, but I assumed it was stress related. Then, I found myself almost falling asleep at the wheel of my car. That was a big wake up event to have happened!

It was then my husband suggested I go to see my GP. I tried a few remedies over the years to stop snoring, including using adhesive strips on the bridge of my nose, but it made no difference. I also had trouble with sinus-itis so assumed it was due to this too.

But the tiredness persisted so reluctantly I made a doctor's appointment, assuming it was a waste of time. 'It's just snoring!' I thought. 'My GP won't do anything.'

I attended the appointment, embarrassed about wasting their time but my GP asked me to take the sleep questionnaire, and immediately she saw I was high risk for sleep apnoea. She suggested going to a sleep clinic. I did not fit any of the usual stereotypes, I was not overweight and I did not drink, etc., but I went for an overnight assessment.

After doing a home sleeping test, it was revealed I stopped breathing 21 times an hour. That meant I had moderate sleep apnoea. What a surprise! I didn't know anything about this condition before and had no idea how dangerous it was.

Immediately I feared I'd have to stop my favourite hobby; flying powered light aircraft. But the Civil Aviation Authority explained if I had treatment and could prove it worked, I was fine to carry on flying. That was a relief, and again, something I didn't expect to happen.

The treatment prescribed was the CPAP machine. I had three motivations to learn to use it: First, my health, I knew I was high risk from strokes and heart issues; second, I had to be fit and well to care for our son; and last, but certainly not least, for my husband. For years he'd been kept awake by my noise!

So, I stuck with wearing the mask, despite it leaking at times, I learned to readjust the mask. I mainly breathe through my mouth so I needed a mask to fit the mouth and nose.

After three nights or so, I slept soundly. The tiredness lifted my energy levels soared. What a gamechanger!

Chapter eleven

The miraculous CPAP machine

CPAP stands for Continuous Positive Airway Pressure and is such a miraculous piece of technology it deserves a chapter in its own right.

Why? Because if CPAP therapy is used properly and regularly, a person's health risks associated with sleep apnoea diminish to those cited as 'normal' in the general population.

Is CPAP basically a 'cure'? Yes, it is on a night-by-night basis!

Love for the machine

Working in the field of sleep medicine is immensely satisfying and it's partly down to the CPAP machine. This therapy changes people's lives – very quickly. There are few disciplines of medicine where a doctor can cure people so fast.

Often within 72 hours of using CPAP our patients have reported all their symptoms vanishing.

From depression to fatigue, from headaches to anxiety, even high blood pressure can be almost instantly reduced.

One of my patients calls his CPAP machine his 'girlfriend who doesn't argue' (sexist, I know!). While others genuinely develop an emotional attachment to this humble device. Why? Because it becomes the guardian of their sleep.

My colleague Shamina's experience is a shining example. She struggled with weight gain after being prescribed pain killers for a bad back. She became depressed, anxious and struggled with her sleep. Eventually she was diagnosed with sleep apnoea after doing a home test. I promised Shamina after one night on CPAP she would feel better. But despite prescribing the treatment to patients herself, she didn't quite believe me. 'Yeah sure,' she laughed.

But in the morning after the first night Shamina reported back.

'I actually felt euphoric. Like I was on drugs. After years of poor sleep, feeling normal is absolutely fantastic. When you feel dreadful, it creeps up slowly and you barely notice it. This must be the reality for a lot of sleep apnoea patients, they don't understand how bad they feel until it stops.'

Shamina got her sleep back and I got a brilliant nurse back. Another happy customer.

CPAP facts: Dr Colin Sullivan, from Australia, invented the CPAP machine in the 1960s. Dr Sullivan helped identify breathing problems in children with sudden infant death syndrome (SIDS) and his research went onto investigate sleep apnoea. He experimented equipment on breeds of dogs including pugs who often experience breathing difficulties before inventing a machine for humans.

The cons of CPAP

Nobody likes the thought of being hooked up to a machine while sleeping. Many people have preconceived ideas about masks and relying on a device. They think it's going to be noisy, uncomfortable to be sleep tethered, or the mask won't fit. Men often worry they'll feel emasculated. This is a particular issue for men, especially those who do not struggle with tiredness despite their sleep apnoea diagnosis. Men can also view mask wearing as being akin to becoming a sick patient in hospital. One patient I had threw his machine in the garage. He couldn't even have it in the house.

It can also be psychologically tricky for the younger man or woman, who is still dating. The worry is that whipping on a sleep mask in the bedroom will be a passion killer. And this could well be the case!

Many patients simply do not like the idea of having to wear a mask to do a basic function like sleep. But I always suggest reframing this image of oneself. I suggest to male patients, who have a sense of humour, to imagine they're Darth Vader or a Top Gun jet pilot! At the end of the joke however is the serious simple message that a CPAP machine saves lives.

Adjusting to sleeping with a mask on can save your life or your health. What could be more worthwhile? Many of us have worn masks for activities like scuba diving or snorkelling and soon get used to them after a few hours. The key is to relax into it and acknowledge you need to use it and think of the extreme benefits involved.

I've had many patients who have still initially refused but eventually realized it isn't as bad as they imagined. I've had patients who point blank refused to try a mask then had two strokes and a heart attack (almost certainly caused by the apnoea) and then returned to ask for a machine after all.

So, I will repeat. CPAP can be a cure-all. The fact is, almost anyone can adapt to sleeping with a mask on, it's just a case of persistence and practise. Many of my patients say they wouldn't be without one or that when they go on holiday it's even the first thing they pack in their suitcase.

How does CPAP work?

Here's the technical bit. There are several types of CPAP machine. The auto CPAP and the fixed pressure CPAP are the most common. Auto CPAP automatically adjusts pressure to meet the patient's breathing need. Whereas the fixed pressure CPAP machine delivers continuous airflow at a pre-set pressure.

There is also a BiPAP (bi-level) machine, which automatically switches between inhalation pressure and a lower exhalation pressure but is for patients with particular needs, such as limited respiratory function. It's far more expensive and rarely prescribed for my patients.

Inside the CPAP machine is an electric motor which acts like a compressor to generate a continuous stream of pressurized air through an air filter into a tube which changes depending on your needs. This filtered air is pushed into the mask that's sealed around your mouth or nose, or both nose and mouth.

Any blockages in a patient's airway are gently opened up by this air stream regulated by a dynamic pressure sensor. This prevents the apnoea, the pause in breath, a bit like when you pump up a tyre to prevent it from being flat.

Thanks to this machine, a patient will no longer need to wake up to start breathing again.

The air pressure in a CPAP machine is set by the sleep clinic. The machine is either supplied by a sleep clinic or bought independently, and you set it yourself. Some machines feature a 'ramp' button (a bit like a snooze button on an alarm clock) which allows the user to gradually increase the pressure until the pre-set pressure is reached. At first it might feel harder to 'exhale' but this feeling often quickly passes. It also has comfort settings of 1, 2, 3 to allow for maximum resistance.

The mask needs to stay on all night in an ideal world. If a patient takes it off by accident at 4am it's not the end of the world. If the mask stays on for the majority of the night, then it will make a big difference to a person's health.

Most patients with OSA will need to use the machine for life. But if this means you end up living a longer, healthier life then every second on a CPAP machine is worthwhile.

CPAP facts: CPAP acts like physio for the lungs and patients with COPD, asthma and other lung conditions have reported marked improvements.

May the CPAP force be with you

I use a mask for my own moderate sleep apnoea. At night, I say to my wife, 'Just going to Darth Vader up!' before a kiss goodnight.

I sleep well, knowing I am doing the best for my health, and she sleeps like a log, knowing I am not going to snore.

There are many mask sizes and shapes, something for everyone. The main type is a triangle shape which fits over the nose and mouth. This can be a good option for those who breath predominantly out of their mouth or have a blockage such as a nose polyp. The mask has a soft flexible cushion that sits snugly on the face. This is the part that can be a challenge to get right. It shouldn't be too tight or too loose otherwise it leaks. Tweaking this at the start is the way to get it right.

Most machines come with a humidifier to warm and moisten the air to make it easier on the throat and nasal passages. In practise however only about 20% of people need this feature. So, unless you need it, do without. It can feel like a faff, cleaning it so you don't get an infection and it can get furred up with hard water too. So, my advice is always start with dry and see if you actually need the humidifier.

The nasal mask covers the whole nose area. This can suit people who move around a lot in their sleep and mainly breathe from their nostrils. The nasal pillow mask is similar except it's two plastic prongs that sit in the nostrils. People who wear glasses and like to read in bed can wear this one comfortably, and it works for men with bushy beards!

There are also masks that fit over the whole face (it's called Fit Life), a bit like a goldfish bowl. This might sound dystopian, but many patients find it comfortable because nothing actually touches the facial area. It's my favourite and reminds me of scuba diving! My colleague, Gill, a sleep specialist nurse, was diagnosed with moderate sleep apnoea, loves this form of mask because she doesn't like the sensation of anything touching her face.

Other types of masks include the oral mask that simply covers the mouth, but this is less popular. Other components of the machine include: mask straps to help keep the mask in place and tubing to link the mask to the machine. At first sight the whole contraption can look unwieldy, and many patients feel anxious or overwhelmed at the idea of using one, especially if they know they'll be on it for life.

But this is where a specialist nurse can save your day (and your life). They're here to patiently help find the right mask for anyone who needs one.

Finding the correct fitting and persevering with tweaking is the key to success. I have met patients who suffer from claustrophobia or who had a near death drowning experience and can't bear their faces to be covered, but there is a design to suit everyone.

Common problems for CPAP machines

In today's world telemonitoring provides online appointments and this is a highly effective way of getting help quickly. You don't have go back and forth to a sleep clinic.

Plus, I can access patient's machines remotely to see online data to ensure the machine is working most effectively. All in all, treating sleep apnoea can be a doddle.

But here are the top six most common issues:

- **Wrong mask shape:** This is the number one reason for CPAP not working.

I often have patients who say: 'I can't wear a mask at night' immediately after diagnosis and I do have to ask if they have tried all 30 shaped masks on the market! Currently there is a huge range and it's growing in style and shapes all the time.

There are many different shape faces, round, square, heart, long, with varying sized noses, and for some people it's trial and error. Depending on what side you sleep, front, back or side sleeping will also affect your choice. I truly believe there is a mask for everyone, even those initially appalled by the idea.

- **Psychology:** This is the second biggest hurdle. Patients have to approach the idea of trying CPAP with an open mind. Everyone is different and what works for one person won't for another.

One patient with sleep apnoea returned to me repeatedly over a six-year period, endlessly trying and failing to sleep with a CPAP machine. But he needed one. He'd already been unwell for years and none of the other treatments were suitable for him. In the end, he came to an appointment and happened to be with his young son who was eight or nine. Suddenly as we discussed options, his boy burst into tears after picking up on our conversation. 'I don't want you to die Dad!' the son cried.

The poor patient went pale and looked at me. There and then he vowed to try and use the CPAP machine again. He went home that day with one and never looked back. He overcame his psychological hurdle for his child, which most of us parents would do. It's all very well if your partner wants you to use a machine but children tug at the heart strings and harden our resolve like nothing else.

- **Dry mouth or nasal congestion:** This can be caused by air flow and a CPAP humidifier is available to help. The warm air opens up the nasal passages making it more comfortable to breathe in. If you're suffering from nasal congestion from an illness a decongestion medication at night is advisable. Although they can only be used for ten days max. If the dryness continues then consider humidification.
- **Air issues:** Sometimes the CPAP machine can cause eye irritation. This happens when the seal of the mask is not tight enough on the face and leaks into the eye. A mask adjustment can rectify this as well as lowering the CPAP pressures. Swallowing air is another issue and some patients can wake up with a bloated stomach. This can be remedied by learning to sleep with your mouth closed (a chin strap can help) or sometimes lying on the left side or propping a pillow behind your back. Occasionally patients report some tightness in the chest, again this is the body adjusting to a new way of breathing.
- **Claustrophobia:** Despite finding a well-fitted mask, some patients report a lingering sensation of claustrophobia if they wear a mask. This usually means you need a different type of mask.
- **Struggling to fall asleep:** Getting used to sleeping with a mask or some kind of device on your face can take time. Ways to acclimatize your body include

practicing wearing the mask during the day for a few hours, building up tolerance to the mask.

For example, one of my colleagues suggests wearing it just for 10 or 20 minutes for the first night and adding blocks of time each night. Sticking to it at the beginning of each night is recommended as this is when we sleep most deeply.

Similarly with the air pressure. Some people find it too harsh to begin with and so reduce the pressure and only gradually increase it over time to a level they feel comfortable with.

Around this time, following my sleep hygiene rules can also help hugely, such as keeping to a regular bedtime, avoiding alcohol and caffeine in the evenings.

At the end of the day (or end of the night!), in an ideal world anyone with sleep apnoea should use their machine all night. But in reality, many patients go off to sleep with the machine then might get up at 5–6am to have a wee, go back and think sod it and don't put it back on. But they are still doing a good 6 hours on therapy and that's doing well.

CPAP facts: Many famous people use CPAP machines. They include:

Former president of the USA, Joe Biden.

Record producer, Quincy Jones.

Pop star, Shaun Ryder.

One of the world's greatest basketball players Shaquille O'Neal.

Star Trek actor William Shatner.

Capital FM DJ Roman Kemp even had his photo taken with his CPAP mask on in *Hello!* magazine.

The scandal of lost time with CPAP

The CPAP machine was invented back in the 1960s but it took until 2008 before NICE recommended the machine as therapy for sleep apnoea, therefore making it easily available to everyone. Why was this? This unnecessary delay is an example of how hierarchical and slow progress in sleep medicine can be.

Back in 1981, a public health doctor called John Sullivan who had no clinical knowledge of CPAP, wrote a report debunking CPAP as therapy even though he didn't review how successfully it was being used around the world. This was published in *The Lancet* which got picked up by NHS commissioning managers who promptly refused to fund CPAP. Once again sleep apnoea began to be viewed as 'just snoring' that didn't deserve funding for treatment.

Decades rolled by, with this Sullivan report cited all over the place to justify not using CPAP. Yet CPAP therapy was being used successfully in countries including America and Australia.

Thankfully, a great guy called John Stradling, an Emeritus Professor of Respiratory Medicine at Oxford decided to challenge the managers who refused funding by providing more evidence for CPAP use. Worldwide data of how brilliantly CPAP was used was collected and eventually this led to a NICE technical assessment in 2008 which concluded that CPAP is the gold standard therapy, after all. This meant the NHS must fund this therapy, which is where we are today.

But still, we lost 27 years where CPAP was side-lined and not funded. Think of how many lives were lost to sleep apnoea due to this poor science. Despite all of Prof Stradling's efforts, in 2019 only about 800,000 (45.71%) of patients are on therapy out of the 1.75 million patients with moderate to severe OSA that would benefit from treatment.

'You can lead a man to CPAP but you can't make him wear the mask.'

Dr Michael Oko

The prize of persistence

I say to all my patients, the rewards of getting back your sleep are so huge, perseverance pays off when it comes to learning to sleep with a mask on. If therapy works, the benefits are life long and can be life changing in ways some people barely dream of.

Case study: Mohammed's story

Mohammed is one of the best examples of someone who didn't give up and utterly transformed his life. Not only did his relationship with his wife and son improve dramatically, but he even changed career, ditching a job he hated for one he loves. He likens using CPAP to 'turning up the colour on a black and white TV.' Here's his story.

Growing up, I was always an outgoing person, and at the age of 25, had lots of hobbies including performing as a clown character called Mojo. But the older I got; the more sleep became an issue for me. However much I slept, I always woke up exhausted.

I worked as a brick layer and builder, so put it down to my busy, stressful job.

By my late 30s, I was really struggling. I had various health issues, including a thyroid problem, so put my exhaustion down to this. My moods grew darker, but I blamed it on not enjoying my work. But the idea of retraining was unthinkable because getting through the day was hard enough.

Then on one occasion I fell asleep in my dinner, a plate of shepherd's pie and gravy! My son and wife woke me up, shouting: 'What's happening to you?' Then the same thing happened at my parent's house, only this time I was sitting on the sofa, and had just been handed a hot cup of tea. The drink landing on my lap soon woke me up.

'What is wrong, son?' Dad asked, worried. This was a good question. I simply didn't know.

My wife had an inkling. She often got woken by my snoring and began to notice I'd stop breathing. Once she timed it and it reached 45 seconds, so she nudged me awake because she feared the worst. She asked me to go

to see the GP numerous times, but I never wanted to. I
didn't expect them to be able to do much.

By aged 40, I looked and felt like a hopeless case.
I had no energy to do anything after work and would
snap at my son if he asked me to play a video game with
him or watch TV. If my wife asked me to go for a meal, I
accused her of being too demanding. I couldn't take any
extra demands on my life, even with loved ones.

I was in bed by 9pm and still woke up exhausted.
Then I'd crave pizza or chocolate for breakfast, desperate
for that quick fix of energy. But at the same time, I felt
flooded with adrenaline, in fight or flight mode. The
mood swings and low energy just ruled my life. As I
got bigger and bigger in size I did less and less with my
family.

By age 41, my wife gave me an ultimatum: 'Go to the
doctors or else!' I didn't fancy finding out what the 'else'
was, so reluctantly went. I told them, 'I am being forced
to come'.

I was annoyed, thinking it a waste of time. But I was
over 18 stone by now, felt and looked dreadful but didn't
want to lose my family too.

Luckily the GP was clued up and suggested sleep
apnoea, so I was put on an NHS waiting list for a sleep
test. I had to wait a long time, but eventually got tested.

They did a sleep study which revealed I was having
63 breath-holding episodes an hour which meant I
had severe sleep apnoea. After being examined it was

revealed I had enlarged tonsils, and it was recommended I use CPAP to open the airways.

Immediately I got a CPAP machine which I didn't fancy using at all. The idea of sleeping with a mask was awful but I knew I needed one to comply with DVLA rules and I needed to drive for my job.

Rather than have the mentality that the treatment wouldn't work, or that I needed something to keep me awake rather than sleep, I gave the masks a go.

I reframed the idea thanks to Dr Oko and thought about Darth Vader, something that appealed to me as a big Star Wars fan. I had to try several different ones, before settling on one that fitted perfectly. It took me a few days and I soon realized I didn't want to sleep without it. The rewards were so instant, I couldn't believe it. My energy levels skyrocketed in days.

Over the next two years it was like someone turning the colour up on a black and white TV.

I stopped craving sugary and fatty foods, so the weight dropped off. I began getting fit again, doing circuit training and martial arts, alongside my son. Then I changed careers and retrained as a teacher. It's a job I'd always wanted to do, but never dreamed it was possible. But I had the energy to go back to college and train. To date I have worked in schools, colleges and even a prison.

I found new hobbies too. I converted an ambulance into a camper van so we could go away as a family. I took my son on a scuba diving holiday, making up for all that lost time when I was too tired for him. I even got a blonde streak put in my hair, just for the fun of it.

I was born in Uganda and am from an East African and Asian background. I have since learned that people from a BAME background are more likely to have sleep apnoea. I believe other family members could benefit from being tested, but it's hard at times to persuade them as they don't like the idea of a mask either.

However, I always say: 'But just look what it did for me!'

I even brought Mojo the Clown back and currently do performances for local charities, bringing a smile to my face and those around me.

Today, I am a completely different person, physically, mentally and emotionally, all because I sleep deeply and properly.

Chapter twelve

Snore off! Other sleep apnoea and snoring treatments

'If love is a sickness, patience is the remedy.'

African proverb

CPAP is not for everyone, but don't despair. Studies show failure rate for CPAP in the UK is 30% although my clinic's failure rate is lower at 20%. Of those 20% of patients who can't use CPAP, we don't give up on them.

The next best option to treat sleep apnoea is the mandibular advancement device (MAD) attachment. This is a device which sits inside the mouth like a rugby player's mouth guard to bring the lower jaw very slightly forward. This moves the tongue's position and opens the airways.

We can monitor its effectiveness by doing a sleep test before it's used and then afterwards. It has about an 80% success rate.

If buying one privately, always get a specialist dentist to make the device – don't try and buy anything online. The alignment is important as over time the device might move your teeth or ruin your jaw joint if the fitting is not correct. It's a bit like choosing glasses for poor eyesight, you need a specialist to get things right or the eyesight will get worse.

Over time the MAD device also degrades as teeth grind onto the attachment, and so regular upkeep and replacement is also necessary.

Case study: Nick's story

One of my sleep apnoea patients, Nick, who didn't want to use a CPAP machine is a real advocate of the MAD device. After his wife threatened to sleep permanently in a spare room, Nick decided to seek help for his snoring.

I was a bit worried myself because I'd wake up in the night, gasping but after my wife complained, I decide to seek help.

Being an ex-military man, who has toured in the Gulf and Afghanistan, I'd become unafraid to speak out if I was suffering from health issues. My past experiences taught me if I needed help, I should get it. Unlike most men I know!

I also felt exhausted in my job as a hospital manager. Often, I felt snappy, irritable and lacked focus. Alongside my problem at home, things had to change.

So, I had a sleep study done and they found sleep apnoea was the issue. Immediately I was offered a CPAP machine but I asked to try a MAD device first. It was agreed I was a good candidate as my issue wasn't that I was overweight, my sleep apnoea was caused by my shape jaw.

On the first night I struggled with using the device. Putting it inside my mouth felt awkward. I wondered how sleep was going to be possible, but I persevered. There is no point in having a sleep study done if you just give up after a few days. I decided to persevere for at least a week. Gradually I got used to it and soon woke up feeling so much more alert and refreshed.

My wife agreed to get back in the bed with me and my days at work felt so much easier too. I couldn't believe such a simple device could transform things so quickly.

Ten years later, I am still using the device every night. It's only if I go out with the lads and come home and forget to wear it do I snore, but my wife soon reminds me to 'get your teeth in' and peace once again is restored.

Last resort: Surgery

What happens if both the CPAP machine and the MAD device don't work? This happens at times, and the CPAP is not for everyone, especially when it comes to treating younger people.

For example, I had a 26-year-old rugby player with sleep apnoea who refused to accept sleeping with a mask for the rest of his life. He was still dating girls and the idea of slipping on a mask after a night together was too much to bear for him.

Luckily, he was a good candidate for surgery, and he successfully had an operation. But for many others surgery won't work or is too risky, for example, if you're 65, overweight and diabetic. It's only an option for young, fit patients who can bounce back post-operatively.

This surgery involves essentially dissecting out the back of the throat, and this obviously cannot be stuck back together again. On evaluating the upper airway, a surgeon will look to see what needs to be removed, that includes parts of the palate, palatine tonsil, lingual tonsil and tongue base.

During the throat surgery there is also the question if a patient will breathe differently under an anaesthetic compared to when they normally sleep. So, deciding on what is causing the turbulence in the throat is a big question for the surgeon. And they are under pressure to find the right answer!

Anyone who has potential sleep apnoea also needs to be diagnosed before surgery. Sleep apnoea patients under anaesthetic need careful monitoring because breath-holding episodes can be fatal. Worst case scenario is embarking on a surgical journey which involves a general anaesthetic, without the anaesthetists knowing whether you will stop breathing or not.

This surgery is not for the faint hearted with a lot of pain and a long recovery time. There are lots of post-op risks including scarring and uncontrollable bleeding and swelling. After the operation the patient will need to stay in the high dependency unit at hospital.

Generally, it was only about 6–7% of patients who actually needed an operation, and this was mainly younger men with big bulky tonsils. Each one had to be justified individually. One of the reasons why the Snoring Disorders Sleep Clinic became so successful is because we quickly also offered unique services that didn't involve surgeries. The NHS commissioners who decided who gets funding liked this as it saved them money too.

There are unscrupulous private health providers which will encourage surgery as a first port of call for snoring and say afterwards, if it doesn't work: 'Oh well at least we gave it a try' so be wary of promises made beforehand.

In my view, no surgery should ever be done unless you really need it. Every single operation comes with risks. Either that it won't work effectively or even worse cause a death.

All surgery to cure snoring and sleep apnoea should be viewed as a last resort, although many of my male patients initially prefer the idea to CPAP and even offer themselves up for it.

Again, it's a predominantly male view to 'fix' the issue fast and with the least amount of fuss. I call it the 'Chop my head off, do whatever it takes, doc' mentality in the mistaken belief it will sort the problem fast. But I always advise extreme caution.

What is the operation's success rate?

After recovery, the success rate of the operations to reduce snoring drops. Interestingly, in around 70% of cases the operation appears successful in the first three months, with less snoring and better-quality sleep reported, but just two years later these dips down to a 50% success rate. Why is this?

It's because post-op patients are in pain, struggle to eat and lose excess weight and so often the apnoea symptoms subside. Then of course patients get better, start eating normally again and the weight piles on and so the sleep apnoea returns, and the operation effectiveness is reduced.

So, the success rate of this operation is the same as the flip of a coin. In good hands this surgery can work, there is no doubt. But it is not fail safe.

Losing weight to cure sleep apnoea

It is possible for obese patients to lose weight and then be cured of sleep apnoea, but it can be a hard path. The issue is a person doesn't know if they became obese due to their sleep apnoea which causes tiredness and the desire to consume more calories. Some patients lose weight, stop CPAP, and then start to feel symptoms again (because they have sleep apnoea whether they're overweight or not) and need to go back on therapy. Once again, all of these individual needs careful monitoring by a health professional.

How do we treat snoring that isn't sleep apnoea?

There are so many wild and wacky antisnore devices on the market, that the choice is mind boggling. From mouth tape to nostril dilators to pillow spray. The market value of snoring products in Europe has been estimated at $0.3 *billion* dollars and that's projected to rise.[79]

Arguably that's because most devices are snake oil and don't work so a new product is always being invented. It can be really confusing but actually if the snoring is not caused by apnoea, then these key things can aid stopping snoring.

Many of the same factors play a role in good sleep hygiene as covered in Chapter thirteen.

1. **Not sleeping on your back:** A lot of people only snore on their back because of the pressure on their airways. Stop this by stitching a tennis ball into the back of your pyjamas.

2. **Nasal congestion:** Use appropriate medication if you're not well but also look at the ventilation in your bedroom. If you don't open the window or door or have some kind of ventilation system (such as a fan or even air con unit) you will get bunged up.

3. **Smoking and drinking:** Both of these activities increase inflammation of the throat and airways which causes snoring.

4. **Allergies:** Food or dust allergies can swell the nasal cavities.

Some snorers swear by nasal strips to open the nostrils, but it really is hit and miss. Remember anything not NICE recommended or prescribed by a medical doctor (and this means they must be registered by the General Medical Council and registered as a specialist if that's what they claim), should be viewed with extreme caution.

There are even groups and associations out there who look very legitimate online with fancy websites or what sounds like legitimate names. Words like 'association' or 'leading UK' can be a red flag unless they're affiliated to a proper medical body. If an 'anti snoring' association looks like a business, it's likely to be a money-making exercise and is best avoided.

Chapter thirteen

What will help *you* to sleep?

'Sleep is the best meditation.'

Dalai Lama[80]

With all the treatment in the world for sleep apnoea, good sleep often can't happen without preparation. Sleep specialists call this 'sleep hygiene' which means preparing ourselves for sleep and considering the conditions where we sleep.

In the hours leading up to going to bed we should wind down and avoid things that make sleep less likely to happen. It means creating a comfortable, relaxing environment that encourages our bodies and minds to 'let go'.

Whatever issue you have, whether it's insomnia or sleep apnoea, how we approach the time to sleep makes a sizable impact on our ability to 'let go' and subsequently our sleep quality.

At the end of a long day, most of us simply fall into bed and hope for the best. I think of sleep as a big pool to dive into. Some of us jump blissfully straight in without hesitation, while others cling to the sides, hesitant. The longer you procrastinate, the harder it can be to jump. Once these hesitancies take hold, it can feel like you're dangling on the edge of the precipice of the pool, increasingly desperate to jump into sleep but unable to. This then causes stressful thoughts to flood in.

'I need to sleep!'

'I have XYZ to do tomorrow and will feel awful if I do not sleep!'

'I only have X hours left to sleep. Oh god!'

And before you know it, you're clinging onto the edge of the pool by fingernails, more desperate than ever to dive in but the 'sleep pool' is rapidly receding.

Being able to sleep is about letting go and not struggling to hold on. This can involve not even consciously 'letting go' (as this stops us for doing so!).

Preparing to sleep with good 'sleep hygiene' helps us to dive straight in, effortlessly, quickly and regularly.

Your mind should welcome sleep when the time comes to go to bed and think nothing more of it. So, when we can't do this, what is happening?

Understanding common sleep disorders

'Nothing tests a marriage more than insomnia or snoring.'

David Linley[81]

All of us sleep badly now and then. It could be because we're stressed about work, exams, relationships, hormone related or due to an underlying health condition. But other factors like the bedroom temperature being too warm, or light pollution, or indeed having a snoring partner can wreck sleep too.

If we sleep badly most of the time, chances are we have a sleep disorder which we will need additional help to overcome.

The most common sleep disorders, aside from sleep apnoea, are as follows:

1. **Insomnia:** This is the inability to sleep or to stay asleep. One in three people in the UK suffers from insomnia. The sleep deprivation makes the following day extremely challenging to function properly and of course tiredness increases hunger, so weight gain is common. It's estimated at least one in ten people have chronic insomnia, which means they struggle to sleep for at least three months.

Insomnia is by far the most common of all sleep disorders and sometimes it can be present alongside sleep apnoea. But how do you know if you have insomnia? Here's a check list.

- Do you have difficulty falling asleep? The average time it takes should be around 10 to 20 minutes, much longer and the answer is yes. Often racing thoughts and negative self-talk stop relaxation.
- Difficulty staying asleep. Do you wake up at night-time and then struggle to drift back off? This can be common in middle age, when a man's prostate is enlarged for example and trips to the loo break sleep cycles. But at other times there might not be a reason for it.

- Do you wake up feeling exhausted? This is a big red flag. Some of us might be night owls and experience low mood in the morning but persistent tiredness is a sign of poor sleep.
- Do you long to nap or sleep during the day?
- Do you struggle with focus and mood issues? This can be a sign of tiredness; however, it becomes so normalized, you might not be conscious of the fatigue!
- In children, is there any difficulty with behaviour or focus at school?

The best medicine for insomnia is CBT, cognitive behavioural therapy (explored in-depth on page 199). Sleeping pills can work in the very short-term but ultimately the psychological reason for the inability to sleep needs dealing with once physical reasons have been ruled out.

2. **Restless leg syndrome:** This is known as Willis-Ekbom disease and is a nervous system condition that makes the legs jerk around, sometimes creating a crawling feeling under the skin. Other causes include secondary disease such as kidney failure or other neurological disorders. In those cases, dopamine altering drugs can be prescribed. It can be common in the third trimester of pregnancy, anaemia is sometimes the culprit so iron supplements may help. If there are no underlying health conditions, stopping smoking and exercising regularly can help the condition. There is growing evidence restless leg syndrome is associated with early signs of dementia.[82]

3. **Parasomnias:** These sleep behaviours can be seen in up to 20% of children and may be REM related (including sleep paralysis), non-REM related (including sleep-walking, night terrors) or other sleep related hallucinations

Rare sleep disorders include:

- **Narcolepsy:** This is a lifelong condition where people can suddenly fall asleep, sometimes without warning, during the day. It can cause a condition known as cataplexy where speech becomes slurred and muscle tone is suddenly lost so a person collapses. This can even be brought on by sudden overwhelming emotions like laughter or tears.

Very rare sleep disorders include:

- **Fatal familial insomnia:** This starts as insomnia but gets progressively worse until the person becomes seriously unwell. Some patients can die after three months of little to no sleep. This is a genetic condition but thankfully as rare as rocking horse manure – only about 50 cases worldwide.

If your GP doesn't ask about sleep, tell them!

If you consistently can't sleep, it's worth visiting a GP to see if you have any underlying health issues.

During doctor appointments GPs often don't ask about sleep.[83] One American study revealed that only 43% of GPs enquire about sleep compared to around 80% who asked about diet and exercise. Sleep might be the best medicine that prevents so many diseases but it's yet to be picked up on the common radar.

There is a voluntary programme in the NHS called Quality and Outcomes Framework (QOF) where medics are given incentives in patient care. For example, it was recognized that taking a patient's blood pressure could help better outcomes, so GPs were incentivized and given a payment for every patient's blood pressure taken. That meant all of a sudden, many patients were offered a blood pressure test whether they asked for it or not!

Perhaps if GPs were requested by QOF to ask about sleep, this might point to better diagnosis where lack of sleep is the cause of the issue.

Once all health disorders have been ruled out (a GP may recommend a blood test) then it's time to examine what's happening in the lead up to bedtime.

The biggest obstacles to sleep

These are the basic sleep saboteurs that makes us hesitant to dive into the pool of sleep – even if we really *want* to. All the factors below will almost certainly cause the hesitancy so learn what they are and decide to avoid them.

- **Not having a routine:** Our internal body clock loves routine. This is how our bodies work at the optimum. Sleeping in late can wreck the following night's sleep. This is why sleeping in at weekends is not a good idea. For example, if you stay up late on a Saturday night and sleep in on the Sunday morning, your sleep will be poor on Sunday night, making the Monday morning blues worse. Stick to the same routine, even if you stay up late, get up at the same time.

- **Caffeine:** Most people will struggle to sleep if they drink cups of tea, coffee or energy drinks in the afternoon. This is because of the time it takes to break down in the body. Not drinking caffeine after midday is a wise decision.

- **Alcohol:** Many of us believe a drink in the evening after work is harmless. But for every unit consumed (that's about a single measure of spirit or 2/3 of as small glass of wine) it takes an hour for the alcohol to be broken down in the body. That means if you drink half a bottle of wine (six units) around 8pm your body is still processing it into the early hours. One study in Finland revealed that *any* amount of alcohol can mess with the REM sleep pattern, with even low amounts decreasing sleep quality by 9%. Moderate alcohol intake (defined as two drinks per day for men and one for women) reduced sleep quality by 24% and heavy alcohol intake reduced sleep quality by nearly 40%.[84] That means booze wrecks sleep, so be mindful of this before opening a bottle.

- **Looking at phones, tablets, video games or other blue lights in the evening:** It's easy to think we can do last-minute emails or catch up with a WhatsApp group after 8pm, but it takes 90 minutes for the effects of blue light to wear off. It might not feel convenient at times (especially in this 24/7 culture, we believe we're 'keeping on top of things' by constantly looking at our phones) but ask yourself: Do I *really* need to respond to that email now? Do you really need to scroll through X (formerly Twitter)/ Facebook/ Instagram after 9pm? The answer is almost always: 'It can wait!'

- **Other forms of light pollution:** Any amount of light can stimulate the pineal gland to reduce the amount of melatonin made. Even a small amount from an extension lead or an alarm clock can mess with our internal clock. Check your room for rogue extension leads or get a black out blind to block lights from outside. A sleep mask can also be a good investment.

- **Trying too hard:** The goal of falling and staying asleep should be to make it as effortless as possible. As soon as conscious panic sets in, our brains go into overdrive. Our aim should be to *not* think too deeply about this natural process. Preparation is advised beforehand but the act of going to bed should happen when you're ready to sleep. If you tend to fall asleep at 11pm don't go to bed at 8pm thinking you're being smart having an early night. The chances are it won't work. If you end up lying in bed, unable to sleep, get up and do something boring like reading a dull book or the ironing. Then when you feel sleepy again, try again. The more you fight to jump into the pool, the further the pool recedes. Only go to bed when you're very tired and ready to sleep.

We are what we eat, and this affects our sleep

Diet has a massive impact on how we sleep. It affects how easily we drop off to sleep and how deeply we sleep.

We all have a gut biome, which is microorganisms that inhabit the gastrointestinal tract and there is evidence to show it affects our health both mentally and physically. One study revealed that over 50% of patients with irritable bowel syndrome had depression, anxiety or sleep problems.[85]

Much of exactly how the gut biome affects our health is still not understood. However, we do know eating and when and what we eat impacts on our ability to sleep.

For example, it's recommended that you avoid eating at least 2–4 hours before bedtime. This is to allow the digestive system to rest too. If you go to bed after a big meal, or even a cup of cocoa, it means your body has an additional job of digesting food rather than resting.

Using a sleep app reveals a lot. Compare what happens to deep sleep episodes if you have eaten just before bedtime compared to not doing so. There will be a big difference in the ability to achieve deep REM.

My advice is this:

- Leave a minimum of 2 hours between your last meal and bedtime.
- Avoid caffeine and alcohol in the evening.
- Avoid too many sugary foods during the day.

Sleep fact: A study from Australia revealed that those eating mostly whole grains, fruit and veg were 19% less likely to suffer from sleep apnoea.[86]

Bedroom habits

'Think in the morning. Act in the noon. Eat in the evening. Sleep in the night.'

William Blake

Considering how many temptations (and expectations!) there are in life that stop us from sleeping, it can feel almost like an act of rebellion to prioritize our sleep.

We don't need a fancy four poster bed or expensive bedding to sleep well, but we do need to think about the room where we sleep. Little things can make a big difference. For example, good ventilation is important.

If a couple shares a bedroom and the window and door is closed, a lot of carbon dioxide will build up over the course of the night. By the morning you'll end up stuffy nosed (which also causes snoring) and a pounding headache.

Temperature is also important. Ideally a room should be around 17–18 degrees Celsius and remain constant, this is because our body heat decreases when we sleep. If the heating kicks in at 5am, it could raise the temperature and wake someone earlier than they wish. Look at the tog of your duvet, is it suitable for winter or summer? Do you need to wear long sleeved pyjamas in bed? Many of us wake up too hot rather than cold.

Would you be better off sleeping alone? I call this 'bedtime divorce' where a couple are in their 40s and 50s, their children have flown the nest, sex drives have dipped, and they have more space so decide to sleep separately. This can suit couples in their comfort years quite happily.

For many it even reignites their sex life as they don't feel the pressure as much *and* they're feeling refreshed by regular sleep.

Consider how a hotel room looks too. The wall colours are always muted browns and creams, furniture is minimal and they always have black out blinds and easy to use temperature controls. These rooms are designed for people to get a good night's kip and nothing else (or sex if you have someone with you!), so compare your bedroom to the simplicity of a hotel room and see what's missing.

Make a buffer zone to relax

Between our busy day and bedtime, we need to create a buffer zone of time to wind down. This could involve chatting with your partner to process events of the day or doing a relaxing, minimally taxing activity, such as watching TV, listening to an audio book, podcast or music. Or it could include very gentle physical activity like stretching or yoga or walking the dog around the block.

In the buffer zone we need to avoid heavy conversations, or excitable books or films that get adrenaline rising. We need to respect this zone as time to unwind from the day's events, to calm anxieties. Occasionally I will play Candy Crush on my phone in the early evening (not too close to bedtime!), to switch off my mind and do something a bit numbing too.

A relaxing activity allows the physical body to encourage the brain to calm down too. This isn't always easy or something that happens naturally, so we have to make a conscious effort to do this. We all have certain likes and dislikes, so try out what works for you.

Whatever you do, avoid drinking alcohol to wind down. It might seem like a fast track to unwinding, but the payoff is poor REM sleep. Anyone who needs a drink before bed, has a problem that needs addressing.

Currently, my favourite way of winding down is listening to an audio book in bed. Favourite author voices include Sandi Toksvig and Stephen Fry because they've got gentle and relaxing tones. There's nothing better than going to sleep with a smile on your face knowing I'll never get to the end of an audio book. I put it on 30 minutes but there is no chance I'll hear the end of it.

Paying to sleep

There's a lot of 'sleep' paraphernalia out there that promises to help us nod off. Some of it people will find helpful (although much will act as a placebo) and be wary of the snake oil again.

Sleep aids on the market including scented pillow sprays, special pyjamas, pillows, eye masks, room scents, weighted blankets, face oils and even a device called a Zeez which claims to mimic brain waves.

I've had great feedback from menopausal patients who have used the Chillow, a chilled pillow that helps with night-time sweats. Sleeping with an air conditioner unit or small fan can also provide control of the room temperature.

Going to sleep peacefully involves psychologically 'letting go' so it makes sense that if we believe we have been given 'help' to let go, it might work. However, there is an ethical question around this when it comes to parting with money for known placebos.

What can be hugely helpful is sleep apps. They can be available for free on your smart phone. None of them are perfect however you can gauge the number of hours of sleep and the depth. It can be a real insight into whether you're achieving the golden 7–8 hours.

They can be handy to experiment with too. Try comparing the results from having a drink or late meal compared to not having it. I know patients who have felt quite competitive with partners, or even with themselves, with trying to 'up' their sleep score.

We know there is nothing as satisfying in life as having had a good night's sleep and seeing the results on an app confirming this can be inspiring.

Sleep fact: The global sleep aids market is tipped to be worth £120 billion by 2030.[87]

Technology that helps me sleep

Some people love gadgets and technology, and I am one of them. As a doctor, I like to feel educated about my health in real life and feedback from gadgets is one way of doing this.

The wearable technology I have includes the Withings Scanwatch 2 which monitors heart health, sleep quality, oxygen levels including breathing disturbances. I also have the sleep mat which monitors heartbeat and breathing rate. I also have their scales and blood pressure monitor. All of my sleep statistics are then easily observed via the Withings app. I think it's a fantastic way of staying up to date in real time on health matters.

But be aware these wearable technologies are only indicative of general health and shouldn't be relied on to self-diagnose conditions. For example, only a medical sleep study with specialized equipment, can determine if medical intervention is needed for a sleep disorder.

The danger of sleeping pills

In the Western world we tend to want to immediately reach for a quick pill to solve a problem. But sleep should not involve pharmacology. End of. Deep restorative sleep cannot be regularly achieved using sleeping tablets. There are no magic sleeping pills on the market which works without any side effects. All of them disrupt the REM cycle.

For short-term insomnia, prescribed drugs can occasionally be helpful if they are used briefly. For example, if someone has suffered a bereavement or job loss, or relationship breakdown or other stressful life event and sleep is disrupted then they can be a temporary solution.

Temazepam is one of the Benzodiazepines and the most common type of prescription sleeping pills. They are generally recommended for short-term use which is less than four weeks. Other prescription sleeping pills include Zoplicone and Zoplidem but of course the side effects are many, including feeling groggy and less focused the next day. They can also make conditions like sleep apnoea worse, simply because the airways become more relaxed and cause blockages.

These medicines work by increasing the strength of your brain's sleep signals that tell your body that it is time to calm down and fall asleep. But they don't promote deep sleep, which of course we need for proper restorative rest.

Long-term drugs don't work because the body becomes resistant to the drugs and needs higher doses to have the same effect.

The most common types of over the counter sleeping aids are antihistamines. Histamine in the brain promotes alertness and when the receptors for histamine are blocked, drowsiness sets in. Companies have marketed diphenhydramine and doxylamine for insomnia under different brand names such as Nytol.

The side effects of antihistamines are not pleasant either. Blurry vision, dry mouth, even constipation can occur and the half-life (the time the medication takes to wear off) is 9–13 hours so the chances of waking up groggy and feeling tired the next day is high.

Other popular medications include melatonin gummies. Melatonin is a hormone produced by the brain in response to darkness. Once it starts to get dark our bodies produce more melatonin which makes us feel sleepy. If we're exposed to light, it can block this.

In America, melatonin is a registered dietary supplement, which means you can buy it anywhere. Officially in the UK, melatonin needs prescription however it is increasingly available to buy on sites like Amazon which is concerning. There are very few long-term studies on the effects of this drug, especially on children. There have been concerns in the US with children overdosing on melatonin gummies with 11,000 cases over three years.

My advice is to only ever give yourself, or your children, drugs which are properly prescribed.

The natural route

Often 'natural' is thought to be less harmful, but this isn't the case. A toadstool is 'natural' but if you ate one, it would kill. There are many herbal (e.g., natural) sleep remedies on the market, such as St John's Wort and Valerian root. They can be taken as pills or teas but be wary of the promises made about restful sleep.

One big risk is 'polypharmacy' where someone takes multiple products not knowing all the side effects and this includes the ingestion of so-called safe and natural products. For example, St John's Wort can interfere with warfarin, a prescribed medicine for anti-blood clotting. If you're taking another prescribed medication alongside natural products, be extra cautious but even if you're otherwise fit and healthy and not taking any medication, these natural supplements can have bad side effects.

The main problem with the 'free market' when it comes to extra vitamins, supplements and sleep aids is that there's not enough data to know how they will interact with or without other drugs.

Plus, if a person has an underlying health issue (perhaps one they don't know about) or is taking multiple drugs at once, it's often a complete unknown about what side effects are.

Without magic sleeping pills what next?

The next port of call is always CBT, cognitive behavioural therapy. This approach is clinically proven to help sufferers of insomnia but involves confronting our personal behaviours and thoughts around sleep.

CBT is essentially the examination of *why* you hesitate to dive into the pool and instead sit on the edge. Our mental approach to sleeping is vital to understand and then challenge. This can be really hard to do, especially if you're over tired and exhausted from years of poor sleep. Finding the headspace to challenge thoughts might feel insurmountable.

But a CBT course is step-by-step and can break down unhelpful and unwanted thoughts replacing them with techniques to control our reactions to them. Studies prove time and again it works so it is worth persisting in trying.

Sleep fact: The longest a person has survived without sleep is 11 days and 25 minutes, a record set by a 17-year-old American in 1963 who was observed as part of an experiment.[88]

Stop off at the sleepstation

Sleepstation is a clinically proven CBT course, designed to combat even severe insomnia and is recommended by NICE and approved by the NHS. This involves an online course using CBTi, which is cognitive behavioural therapy for insomnia in particular and is personalized to the user who fills in a sleep diary.

The course is available to some people on the NHS, or it costs £260. However, through the website you can be offered a grant for £135 which brings the cost down for a nine-week course.

Over the past decade Sleepstation have analysed over a million sleep diaries. The team have a large body of evidence, based on over 100 randomized controlled trials for CBTi being an effective and long-lasting treatment for 50–70% of patients. Their website states that 'CBT takes longer than drugs to produce sleep improvements, but these improvements are sustained over time'.[89]

Once a user has signed up, they complete a weekly sleep diary, and then online techniques are tailored to each person. Some of them are very simple but effective, such as 'thought blocking' techniques. This involves replacing thoughts with a single word or giving specific advice to a patient. For example, many people with sleep disorders go to bed earlier to try and get extra sleep but it can be helpful to stay up later than usual to make sure your body and mind is even more tired. Avoiding naps in the daytime is also often recommended. Additionally, Sleepstation provide online doctors for advice and sleep tips that are sent regularly via email.

Many people who try CBT and say it doesn't work, often have missed out steps or not followed it as advised. For others, particularly those who have serious mental health problems, CBT is not advised, but these questions are covered at the start.

If after trying CBT sleep remains a difficulty, then getting a referral to a sleep clinic is the next best step to see if you have an underlying problem.

The most important factor in dealing with all sleep issues is persistence. It can feel so easy to slip into bad habits such as having a few glasses of wine or relying on a medication like Benadryl to help you drop off. But this wrecks the chances of much needed REM depth. High-quality restorative sleep is a life changer and worth every effort involved to attain regularly. Not just for your sake and your health but for loved ones around you.

Chapter fourteen

Busting sleep myths – what's true or false?

'There is a time for many words, there is also a time for sleep.'

Homer[90]

In 2023 it was reported that Google searches for the word 'sleep' reached an all-time high, which indicates the general population is finally waking up to the importance of sleep.[91] We all need to sleep better, and education is needed.

With so much confusing information out there about sleep and snoring, I hope this book clears much of the fact from the fiction.

To end this book, we look at the common myths busted one question at a time.

1. **'I am used to not getting much sleep and my body has adapted.' True or false?**
   False!

   The body doesn't adapt to lack of sleep, it's more likely the patient has got used to feeling like hell. The scale of 'tiredness' (or 'excessive sleepiness' as the DVLA likes to describe it) is *very* hard to assess for an individual. For example, if you're a new mum and waking every hour, chances are you know you're tired and can describe the effect on your body. This is because it's a relatively sudden new development. You might have slept well before the baby and suddenly experience broken nights after the birth.

However, if you've had sleep apnoea for years, it's possible the symptoms have become 'normalized'. If you've always got a headache in the mornings or feel exhausted by the afternoon, it can be easy to dismiss. If you're used to a low mood, it's hard to know what feeling positive is like.

No human body 'adapts' successfully to a lack of sleep. The physiological damage will be done.

2. **'Resting with your eyes closed is as good as sleep.' True or false?**
False!

Nothing beats deep restorative sleep where deep sleep and REM levels are achieved. No sleeping pill or meditation or short restful period. We need proper deep sleep, and this is much more likely to be achieved by following sleep hygiene rules.

3. **'Loud snoring runs in our family and never did anyone harm.' True or false?**
Well, it *could* be true.

Some loud snoring is harmless, and snoring can run in families due to similar sized and shaped bodies or behaviours. However, loud snoring and sleep apnoea also runs in families because of our physiology or similar lifestyles too. For example, excess weight tends to run in families (not only due to genetics but also diets we learn to eat) and this is more likely to cause snoring and sleep apnoea. Also, a recessed jaw can cause sleep apnoea so if you've inherited such a trait from your parent, it can cause snoring and sleep apnoea.

Many people from previous generations will have suffered from undiagnosed sleep apnoea and died from causes related to it and nobody will have known. For example, if your parent died of a heart attack, stroke, cancer or diabetes complications *and* they snored it's very possible they may have had sleep apnoea which tragically contributed to the development of their illness. In most cases from the early noughties backwards, most people won't have been diagnosed with OSA so whether a loved one's snoring contributed to their final illness cannot be confirmed.

4.   **'Having a night cap helps me drop off and sleep better.'**
     True or false?
     True and false!

It is true that alcohol can make us feel sleepy and so gives the sensation that it helps us to drop off to sleep more easily.

But studies have revealed even one drink, and doesn't matter what it is, wine, beer, whisky, brandy, a hot toddy (yes even those traditional nightcap drinks we convince ourselves do no harm) can interrupt the deep restorative REM we need. So, it is false that alcohol helps us to sleep 'better'. Anyone who feels they need a drink to get to sleep should seek medical advice.

5. **'Having a quick afternoon nap makes up for a bad night's kip.' True or false?**

    True-ish!

    If you haven't slept well the previous night, a daytime nap can certainly help with energy levels and focus on work. However, it should be restricted to a short nap of around 20 minutes and not late in the afternoon. I always advise patients to nap if they feel the need to and not feel guilty about it. Sleep should always be kept a big priority for our mental and physical health.

6. **'Getting rid of excess energy by exercising before bed is always a good idea.' True or False?**

    False!

    Exercising vigorously within 2 hours before bedtime can increase adrenaline and cortisol levels which inhibit our ability to switch off and prepare for a good night's sleep. It's better to exercise during the day, especially getting natural day light at the same time. This can aid restful deep sleep.

7. **'You can get too much sleep.' True or false?**

    True!

    Studies have shown that oversleeping can be as much of an issue as not getting enough sleep. People who sleep for over 10 hours were more likely to have psychiatric issues or higher body mass index than those who slept shorter hours.[92]

8. **'It's normal to struggle to sleep the older you get.' True or false?**

True!

Many people experience insomnia or sleep issues as they age, especially women. This can be due to a range of reasons from perimenopause symptoms, childcare, work stresses and strains or illnesses. We all experience insomnia at some point in our lives. It's also possible we will have less sleep the less active we become too. However, getting less sleep when we're older should not be viewed as an inevitable part of ageing because it still has a detrimental impact on our lives.

It is not true to say older people 'need less sleep'. They don't. We should continue to aim for 7–8 hours of sleep a night. If you're experiencing early awakening it could be to do with other illness, stress or what you're eating and drinking late into the night. Lifestyle changes can be tweaked for us to attain those golden hours we need as we age. The importance of getting good sleep does not diminish as we age.

9. **'Catching up on lost sleep at the weekends is energizing.' True or false?**

False!

It can feel temporarily good to have a lie in on a Saturday, but it's false to say that you're 'catching up on lost sleep'. Everyone needs regular 7–8 hours of sleep and our body clock thrives off routine. We cannot sleep badly all week and then make up for it on a Saturday and Sunday morning. In fact, it will mess with our body circadian rhythms. For example, if you sleep in on a weekend, you are likely to struggle to drop off at your normal bedtime on Sunday evening and make Monday morning even harder to deal with!

10. **'Sleeping gives your body and brain a total rest.' True or false?**
False!

If you look at an EEG of the brain during the time asleep it lights up in ways totally unexpected. Sleep is a very active process and much of it remains a mystery to scientists. What we do know however is that deep sleep triggers the glymphatic system which flushes cleans the brain debris.

Our brains do not rest when we're fast asleep. The exact opposite happens.

11. **'The idea of needing a CPAP mask stops most people from having a sleep test.' True or false?**
Probably true!

The resistance to the idea of needing a sleep mask is definitely common. Why would *anyone* like the idea of sleeping with a mask unless they have to? However, the reality is that the vast majority of my patients are able to adapt to wearing one and quickly. Around 80% of my patients who need CPAP, are able to use it regularly. Plus, it saves lives and stops loud snoring. The benefits outweigh the cons of the preconceived ideas. Most people are pleasantly surprised at how easy they are to adapt to wearing and how much better they feel for it. Don't knock it until you try it!

12. **'Wearing a CPAP mask can change your life for the better overnight.' True or false?**
    True!

    I usually suggest to patients to allow for it to work within 72 hours if it's fitted correctly. That means they can look forward to deeper sleep, improved energy levels and better focus during the day. I have had patients say it has changed their life overnight too.

13. **'I will use CPAP until my breathing adapts and then I can stop using it.' True or false?**
    False!

    Most people need CPAP for life. In some circumstances people might lose weight and if this happens it can naturally reduce their apnoea and need for CPAP.

14. **'Children who snore grow out of it.' True or false?**
    Not true or false!

    We don't know as there isn't the data to prove or disprove this theory. What we do know is that tonsil size can reduce over time, however the damage of the lack of sleep due to the apnoea could have been done by then.

15. **'Men snore more than women.' True or false?**
    True!

    But also, increasingly women are coming forward to get a sleep test done due to their concerns about snoring. With rising levels of obesity in both men and women, we can expect sleep apnoea numbers to rise.

16. **'Loud snoring is always a sign of sleep apnoea.' True or false?**

False!

It isn't always. But it needs checking out because loud snoring is a common sign of OSA and this needs investigation.

17. **'I don't feel tired so I can't have sleep apnoea.' True or false?**

False!

Some patients have OSA and surprisingly do not feel any tiredness, but as previously discussed how tired you are is a subjective thing!

18. **'The reason why sleep isn't a priority for many doctors is because other medical issues are more important.' True or false?**

False!

Lack of sleep or consistent poor sleep is proven to have devastating impacts on many areas of our bodies and mental health. If you consistently lack sleep the statistics prove you face developing chronic disease. The medical world however is resistant to change and sleep science is still in its infancy. For a peer reviewed paper to be made about a certain subject it costs a lot of time and money. Sleep is woefully underinvested over the years compared to many disciplines such as cancer or heart disease. This needs to change. This is happening. But it could and should happen faster.

19. **'My friend only needs 5 hours sleep and he's fine.' True or false?**

False!

Well, he might tell you he's fine but there are likely to be short- and long-term consequences for little sleep. The data is clear that consistently sleeping less than 7–8 hours a night regularly has a negative impact on our health and overall mortality rates. There will always be an exception to this rule if we consider the bell curve of humanity. But the number of people who need less sleep will be tiny and the chances are it's not going to be your friend.

My manifesto for raising awareness of OSA

To end this book, I include a manifesto which I have developed with my long-term college Professor, Ram Dhillon, for ENTUK and the All-Party Parliamentary Working Group on OSA. I would like to raise awareness of sleep apnoea, educate people on health risks and make finding treatment for OSA easier. It's a (not-so-) silent killer, that needs urgently addressing.

Let me remind you of the stark statistics.

The latest figures show 8.7% of men and 5.6% of women between the ages of 30–75 in the UK have obstructive sleep apnoea (OSA). This is around 4 million individuals with OSA which makes sleep apnoea as common as diabetes. Around 1.75 million of these people will have moderate or severe OSA.

OSA mainly affects men, postmenopausal women and the BAME community. Anyone with sleep apnoea faces significant risks to their health. They are twice as likely to become obese, and 1.5 times more likely to have a stroke or develop cancer. Around 50% of people with diabetes also have sleep apnoea and 40% of those with dementia have it, but in almost all cases will not know it.

According to Professor John Stradling in 2019 we are only treating 800,000 out of 1.75 million (45.71%) people with moderate to severe OSA with CPAP that would benefit from therapy. This means we need to more than double our current capacity nationally! For example, in Lincolnshire, where I work, we still have a very long way to go as we are only treating about 4,700 patients out of an anticipated 35,000 who should be on therapy, or about 1 in 7.

The cost to our society is gigantic but also little understood. Not only the economic cost, with road traffic accidents caused by excessive sleepiness, but also the medical costs of treating these chronic conditions caused by OSA.

A national campaign to raise awareness began in January 2024 with an All-Party Parliamentary Group (APG) of Lords, MPs, Kath from OSA charity Hope2Sleep, other experts and members of NHS and Primary Care Teams and of course, me.

We cannot expect miracles to happen within a strained NHS system so we must be realistic in our aims. As a surgeon, who has set up a clinic from nothing, I understand the process and bottlenecks in provision of a good sleep disorder service. As part of my journey, I have learned to cut through the red tape and managerial procrastination that impedes efficient delivery of service. However, it's creating awareness that will save people's lives. We all know the saying 'prevention is better than a cure' and regarding sleep apnoea it's a perfect description. By treating (and in many cases pretty much curing) sleep apnoea we prevent so much unnecessary suffering from disease and untimely deaths.

Here are the changes I would like to see:

1. **Increase public awareness of sleep apnoea:** The APPG aims to hold high level parliamentary talks to

help promote understanding of OSA. I aim to offer every single person sitting in the House of Lords a screening for sleep apnoea.

2. **Promote awareness within the NHS:** We hope to spread the word to medics, GPs and consultants. We want to encourage doctors to ask patients questions about their sleep when it's appropriate. With increased medical awareness, more patients can be offered sleep tests. Likewise, nurses should be trained in setting up sleep machines such as CPAP therapy if a patient needs this.

3. **Increase awareness within the childcare sector:** Give information to schools or nurseries or to health visitors to help spot the signs of OSA in children.

4. **Screen all perimenopausal women and pregnant women:** They could be screened with a modified Stop Bang form. This could help reduce the mass exodus of postmenopausal women from the workforce. When I triage referrals, I add one point each for diabetes, stroke, heart attack or dementia.

5. **Completely redesign OSA pathways and priorities:** To do this there are several quick wins that can be deployed. Here are my suggestions in detail:

   a. **Convince the private insurance market that it is bad for business not to recognize sleep apnoea:** Instead, they should follow NICE guidance and pay for diagnosis *and* treatment, as private insurers in the US do. This would open treatment for about 22% of the population (number of adults with private medical insurance has jumped

from 12% in 2019 as a result of the NHS struggling to deliver patient care). The private insurers
could also potentially save money on their policies as evidence suggests that they will save 50%
on health costs within two years! Surely this is a
quick win–win?

b. **All current NHS sleep clinics should replace
face-to-face with virtual consultations for
efficiency:** I can get through roughly twice the
number of patients in the same time as a face-to-
face clinic and my patient satisfaction is >95%.

Sleep kits can also be easily delivered to a home too
which also means patients no longer need to make round
trips to the clinic. Any NHS business managers reading
please take note it costs at least £400 per 4-hour clinic
for room space. Plus, the patients must pay for travel and
parking for something that could be completed with a quick
phone call!

Face-to-face appointments also create an unnecessary
high impact on the environment due to the number of car
journeys involved. We do about 17,000 consultations per
year and about 80% of patients are fully compliant and happy
with their therapy despite being remote appointments. It is
estimated that the NHS contributes about 5.4% of greenhouse
gases in the UK. We need to clamp down on clinics that do
not need to be attended in person.[93]

How long would a normal round trip by car take to attend a clinic at Pilgrim or Johnson hospitals?

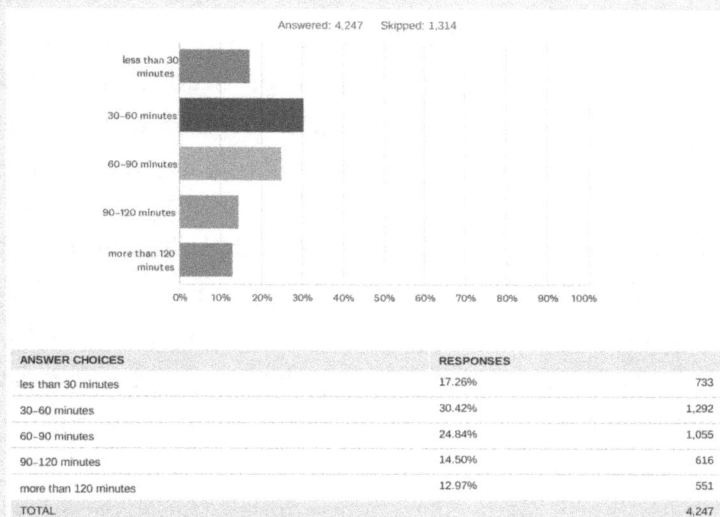

Answered: 4,247   Skipped: 1,314

ANSWER CHOICES	RESPONSES	
les than 30 minutes	17.26%	733
30–60 minutes	30.42%	1,292
60–90 minutes	24.84%	1,055
90–120 minutes	14.50%	616
more than 120 minutes	12.97%	551
TOTAL		4,247

c. **Make sleep clinic appointments more efficient,** including:

   i. Move all routine and compliant patients to annual appointments. The slots freed up should be allocated to the 20% or so that are struggling with therapy.

   ii. Follow ups should be intelligence driven using modern technology to anticipate that a patient is struggling with therapy.

   iii. No patient should be asked to return their CPAP kit to the local hospital if they move out of area. This is a wasteful, immoral and disgraceful practice that I see with patients relocating to Lincolnshire often left without therapy when their old local clinic instructs them to return all equipment. This practice has not been thought through. What would be the legal repercussions of this action if a patient had a stroke or heart attack? This wastes resources, duplicates care and deprives the patient of what could be lifesaving therapy!

6. **They are clear guidelines from NHS England: Who pays document NHS England » Who Pays?** Essentially the Integrated Care Board (ICB) that you currently live in before you move has to pay the costs and sort it out with the new ICB of the postcode you will move to. This should not delay your care!

   a. ICBs need to be reminded they have a legal right to NICE approved treatments in a reasonable timescale under the NHS constitution. They have a duty to resource and plan for provision of these services. They should all be held accountable and league tables must be published monthly as they do for other NHS waiting times.

   b. A tracker of every patient referred needs to look at bottlenecks in the system. This should include:

      i. Time from GP referral to first appointment in clinic (often patients officially come off the waiting list at this point!). All routine appointments should complete pathway and be on therapy within 18 weeks: Urgent two to three weeks; HGV drivers or other vigilant roles weeks; Inpatients needing discharge home should be less than one week.

ii. Time from clinic to sleep study.

iii. Time from sleep study to receiving therapy.

7. **Finally, the NHS should ring fence funding for future research:** I would like to approach big tech companies directly for funding into sleep deprivation research. Working collaboratively with big tech companies makes sense as they hold the 'big data' on our use of devices and technology. It's an ambitious idea, but one all of society could benefit from.

Endnotes

[1] Alsaif, S.S., Kelly, J.L., Little, S., Pinnock, H., Morrell, M.J., Polkey, M.I., and Murphie, P. (2022) Virtual consultations for patients with obstructive sleep apnoea: A systematic review and meta-analysis. *European Respiratory Review*, 31(166): 220180. doi: 10.1183/16000617.0180-2022.

[2] https://pubmed.ncbi.nlm.nih.gov/30597439/

[3] Nunn, C.L. and Sampson, D.R. (2018) Sleep in a comparative context: Investigating how human sleep differs from sleep in other primates. *American Journal of Physical Anthropoly*, 166(3): 601–612.

[4] https://quotefancy.com/quote/1001873/William-Golding-Sleep-is-when-all-the-unsorted-stuff-comes-flying-out-as-from-a-dustbin

[5] www.southampton.ac.uk/medicine/news/2020/02/18-link-between-brain-waste-and-alzheimers.page

[6] www.tandfonline.com/doi/abs/10.1179/016164106X130506

[7] www.brainyquote.com/quotes/anthony_burgess_136600

[8] www.sleepapnoea.org/central-sleep-apnoea/

[9] www.ncbi.nlm.nih.gov/pmc/articles/PMC2952752/#:~:text=Snoring%20is%20common%20in%20the,of%20men%20reporting%20habitual%20snoring.&text=It%20is%20the%20most%20common,%25%20to%2095%25%20of%20patients

[10] www.independent.co.uk/voices/commentators/sloane-crosley/sloane-crosley-perhaps-my-neighbours-are-trapped-under-some-very-weighty-pieces-of-furniture-ndash-a-girl-can-dream-2236949.html

[11] www.brainyquote.com/quotes/alfred_hitchcock_100225

[12] www.ncbi.nlm.nih.gov/pmc/articles/PMC5836788/

[13] Redline, S., Tishler, P.V., Hans, M.G., et al. (1997) Racial differences in sleep-disordered breathing in African-Americans and Caucasians. *American Journal of Respiratory and Critical Care Medicine*, 155: 186–192.

[14] Ancoli-Israel, S., Klauber, M.R., Stepnowsky, C., et al. (1995) Sleep-disordered breathing in African American elderly. *American Journal of Respiratory and Critical Care Medicine*, 152: 1946–1949.

[15] www.ncbi.nlm.nih.gov/pmc/articles/PMC6733415/#:~:text= The%20physiologic%20changes%20of%20pregnancy,snoring%20 in%20the%20third%20trimester.&text=Among%20obese%20 pregnant%20women%2C%2015%25–20%25%20have%20OSA, (BMI)%20and%20other%20comorbidities

[16] www.ncbi.nlm.nih.gov/pmc/articles/PMC5323064/

[17] https://err.ersjournals.com/content/28/154/190030

[18] https://pubmed.ncbi.nlm.nih.gov/15781100/

[19] www.cell.com/current-biology/fulltext/S0960-9822(23)00156-2

[20] https://pubmed.ncbi.nlm.nih.gov/32780010/

[21] www.nebraskamed.com/COVID/want-to-support-your-immune-system-better-sleep-on-it#:~:text=First%20of%20all%2C%20 more%20sleep,to%20develop%20a%20viral%20infection

[22] www.cancerresearchuk.org/health-professional/cancer-statistics/ statistics-by-cancer-type/breast-cancer/risk-factors

[23] Dehesh, T., Fadaghi, S., Seyedi, M., et al. (2023) The relation between obesity and breast cancer risk in women by considering menstruation status and geographical variations: A systematic review and meta-analysis. *BMC Women's Health*, 23: 392. https:// doi.org/10.1186/s12905-023-02543-5

[24] Zhang, R. et al. (2014) A circadian gene expression atlas in mammals: implications for biology and medicine. *Proceedings of the National Academy of Sciences of the United States of America*, 111(45): 16219–16224. doi: 10.1073/pnas.1408886111.

[25] www.nih.gov/news-events/nih-research-matters/time-day-can-be-critical-chemotherapy

[26] https://epworthsleepinessscale.com/sleepiness/

[27] https://ftp.cdc.gov/pub/Health_Statistics/NCHS/NHIS/SHS/2014_SHS_Table_A-18.pdf

[28] www.theguardian.com/society/2012/nov/04/men-failing-seek-nhs-help

[29] www.dailymail.co.uk/sciencetech/article-11969601/One-10-frazzled-Britons-considered-leaving-partner-SNORING-study-finds.html

[30] https://quotefancy.com/quote/861519/Mark-Twain-There-aint-no-way-to-find-out-why-a-snorer-can-t-hear-himself-snore

[31] Look After Yourself! Micky Flanagan: Back in The Game Live. YouTube. www.youtube.com/watch?v=jS4u-cqEgR0

[32] wendyatthewendyhouse.co.uk

[33] www.thecut.com/2014/10/romantic-gestures-according-to-amy-poehler.html

[34] www.gov.uk/government/calls-for-evidence/womens-health-strategy-call-for-evidence/outcome/results-of-the-womens-health-lets-talk-about-it-survey

[35] www.center4research.org/everything-is-designed-for-men-even-drugs/

[36] https://err.ersjournals.com/content/28/154/190030

[37] www.preeclampsia.org/the-news/research/does-sleep-apnoea-increase-risk-for-preeclampsia

[38] Facco, F.L. (2015) LB2: Prospective study of the association between sleep disordered breathing and hypertensive disorders of pregnancy and gestational diabetes. *American Journal of Obstetrics and Gynaecology*, 212(1): S424–S425. doi: 10.1016/j.ajog.2014.11.028.

[39] https://publications.parliament.uk/pa/cm5803/cmselect/cmwomeq/91/report.html

[40] https://committees.parliament.uk/oralevidence/9793/html/

[41] www.brainyquote.com/quotes/frederick_douglass_201574

[42] Powell, S., et al. (2010) Paediatric obstructive sleep apnoea. *BMJ*, 340. doi: https://doi.org/10.1136/bmj.c1918.

[43] https://news.sky.com/story/shaun-ryder-i-think-ive-had-coronavirus-but-im-fine-ive-been-isolating-for-years-11965892

[44] https://ndss.org/resources/sleep-down-syndrome#:~:text=Children%20with%20Down%20syndrome%20are,the%20rest%20of%20the%20population

[45] https://stackoverflow.selfgrowth.com/articles/words-of-wisdom-laozi?no_redirect=true

[46] https://pubmed.ncbi.nlm.nih.gov/37087382/

[47] www.ons.gov.uk/peoplepopulationandcommunity/populationandmigration/populationprojections/bulletins/nationalpopulationprojections/2020basedinterim

[48] Andrade, A.G., Bubu, O.M., Varga, A.W., and Osorio, R.S. (2018) The relationship between obstructive sleep apnea and Alzheimer's disease. *Journal of Alzheimer's Disease*, 64(s1): S255–S270. doi: 10.3233/JAD-179936.

49 www.dailymail.co.uk/news/article-1201897/Brown-needs-sleep-run-country-properly-says-aide-Tony-Blair.html

50 www.brainyquote.com/quotes/jackie_chan_464598

51 www.statista.com/topics/6188/coffee-market-in-the-uk/#topicOverview

52 www.southampton.ac.uk/news/2017/11/coffee-health-benefits.page

53 https://britishcoffeeassociation.org/coffee-consumption/

54 www.brainyquote.com/quotes/frankie_boyle_1076756

55 https://durham-repository.worktribe.com/output/1167893/

56 www.bda.uk.com/resource/energy-drinks-and-young-people.html

57 www.ncbi.nlm.nih.gov/pmc/articles/PMC8507757/

58 www.theguardian.com/business-to-business/2017/dec/04/clocking-off-the-companies-introducing-nap-time-to-the-workplace

59 www.addictioncenter.com/drugs/phone-addiction/

60 www.theguardian.com/global/2021/aug/22/how-digital-media-turned-us-all-into-dopamine-addicts-and-what-we-can-do-to-break-the-cycle

61 www.independent.co.uk/advisor/vpn/screen-time-statistics; www.healthline.com/health/what-is-blue-light#takeaway

62 www.cbc.ca/news/canada/british-columbia/bc-supreme-court-class-action-epic-games-fortnite-1.6784958

63 www.news-medical.net/news/20230501/Excessive-digital-technology-use-is-associated-with-reduced-sleep-quality-regardless-of-environmental-and-genetic-factors-study-finds.aspx

[64] www.birmingham.ac.uk/news-archive/2019/researchers-reveal-brain-connections-that-disadvantage-night-owls

[65] www.nimh.nih.gov/health/publications/the-teen-brain-7-things-to-know

[66] www.theguardian.com/education/2022/sep/14/california-later-school-start-times-law-teens-sleep

[67] www.sciencedaily.com/releases/2020/02/200218125312.htm

[68] www.brainyquote.com/quotes/tom_hodgkinson_527558

[69] AAA Foundation for Traffic Safety in the US.

[70] The American Academy of Sleep Medicine.

[71] www.ncbi.nlm.nih.gov/pmc/articles/PMC5627640/

[72] www.personneltoday.com/hr/employees-accident-mistake-tiredness-at-work/

[73] https://post.parliament.uk/research-briefings/post-pn-0586/

[74] bma_fatigue-sleep-deprivation-briefing-jan2017.pdf

[75] www.theguardian.com/society/2017/jul/06/half-of-junior-doctors-having-accidents-or-near-misses-after-night-shifts

[76] www.hse.gov.uk/humanfactors/topics/fatigue.htm

[77] www.ncbi.nlm.nih.gov/pmc/articles/PMC5627640/

[78] https://pubmed.ncbi.nlm.nih.gov/35830509/

[79] www.marketdataforecast.com/market-reports/europe-anti-snoring-devices-market

[80] www.youtube.com/watch?v=llLtYd_ZSzA

[81] www.brainyquote.com/topics/snoring-quotes

[82] https://alzres.biomedcentral.com/articles/10.1186/s13195-023-01191-z

[83] www.ncbi.nlm.nih.gov/pmc/articles/PMC5102393/

[84] www.medicalnewstoday.com/articles/321731#Even-low,-moderate-drinking-impairs-sleep

[85] www.ncbi.nlm.nih.gov/pmc/articles/PMC6290721/#:~:text= There%20is%20considerable%20evidence%20showing,microbiome %2Dgut%2Dbrain%20axis

[86] www.theguardian.com/society/2024/feb/21/plant-based-diet-cuts-sleep-apnoea-risk-by-a-fifth-research-shows

[87] www.cim.co.uk/content-hub/editorial/how-sleep-fatigued-consumers-are-shaking-up-the-wellbeing-market/

[88] www.newscientist.com/question/how-long-can-you-go-without-sleep/

[89] www.sleepstation.org.uk/evidence/

[90] www.allgreatquotes.com/

[91] https://apple.news/AC8jW9tPvSneriIQvbX8ZVg

[92] www.ncbi.nlm.nih.gov/pmc/articles/PMC4165901/

[93] The NHS produces 5.4% of the UK's greenhouse gases. How can hospitals cut their emissions? NHS. *The Guardian*. www. theguardian.com/society/2019/sep/18/hospitals-planet-health-anaesthetic-gases-electric-ambulances-dialysis-nhs-carbon-footprint

Index

A quick word from Practical Inspiration Publishing...

We hope you found this book both practical and inspiring – that's what we aim for with every book we publish.

We publish titles on topics ranging from leadership, entrepreneurship, HR and marketing to self-development and wellbeing.

Find details of all our books at: www.practicalinspiration.com

Did you know...

We can offer discounts on bulk sales of all our titles – ideal if you want to use them for training purposes, corporate giveaways or simply because you feel these ideas deserve to be shared with your network.

We can even produce bespoke versions of our books, for example with your organization's logo and/or a tailored foreword.

To discuss further, contact us on info@practicalinspiration.com.

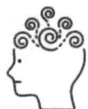

Got an idea for a business book?

We may be able to help. Find out more about publishing in partnership with us at: bit.ly/PIpublishing.

Follow us on social media...

@PIPTalking

@pip_talking

@practicalinspiration

@piptalking

Practical Inspiration Publishing